Chad Prince, MSPT

Physical Therapy Career & Salary Guide

Avoid the Income Ceiling and Put Your Career in the FASTLANE

**Published in the United States by
UELadder, LLC
Independent Publishers
www.UELadder.com/pages/PTBook**

Copy Editor: Beth Balmanno
Content Editor: Stephen Huntsman

Copyright 2016 by William Chad Prince
Researched and written by William Chad Prince

All rights reserved. Without limiting the rights under the copyright reserved above, no part of this publication may be reproduced, stored in, or introduced into a retrieval system, or transmitted in any form or by any means (electronic, mechanical, photocopying, recording, or otherwise) without prior written permission.

For permission requests, please contact:
cp@chadprince.com

Disclaimer

This is a work of nonfiction. The events and experiences detailed herein are all true and have been as faithfully rendered as the author can represent them, to the best of his abilities. Some names, identities, and circumstances have been changed in order to protect the privacy and/or anonymity of the various individuals involved.

Please note: this book represents the personal opinions of the author. Chad Prince does not engage in tax, legal or accounting services. This material has been prepared for informational purposes only, and is not intended to provide, and should not be relied on for tax, legal or accounting advice. Before making any business decisions please consult a licensed professional.

TABLE OF CONTENTS

INTRODUCTION 4
INITIAL EVALUATION 7
Part 1 Fill Your Toolbox 11
  Chapter 1 Find Your Why 12
  Chapter 2 Build an Affirmation Statement 17
  Chapter 3 Create Daily Routines 23
  Chapter 4 30-Day Challenge 26
Part 2 The State of PT Salaries Today 27
  Chapter 5 How Much Do PTs Make? 28
  Chapter 6 The Pros of Physical Therapy 36
  Chapter 7 Health Care Challenges 40
  Chapter 8 Physical Therapy Business Models 44
  Chapter 9 The Cons of Physical Therapy 53
Part 3 The First Decade 57
  Chapter 10 Crawl, Walk, Run 58
  Chapter 11 Hitting the Ceiling 68
RECERTIFICATION 76
Part 4 Raise the Ceiling 77
  Chapter 12 Slowlane and Fastlane 78
  Chapter 13 Opportunities in Standard PT Practice 87
    PRN Work 89
    Specialization and Certification 93
    Private Practice Outpatient Clinics 97
    Niche Markets 102
    Solo Clinics 111
    Minority Ownership Clinic 123
    Contract Therapy Services 126

Chapter 14 *Opportunities in Supporting PT Industries* 139
    Educational Products 144
    Live Speaker Continuing Education 148
    Online Continuing Education Provider 151
    Online Platform for Continuing Education 157
    Self-Publishing 166
    Physical Therapy Business Consulting 173
    Physical Therapy Business Education 177
    Physical Therapy Software Services 184
    Physical Therapy Product Creation 201

Part 5 Conclusion 219
Chapter 15 *Concluding Thoughts and Parting Business Advice* ... 220
DISCHARGE SUMMARY 235
Bonus Materials 237

*This book is dedicated to my wife, Michele,
and to our two daughters, Mileah and Cara,
with all of my love.*

*Special thanks goes to all of the gracious therapists
who answered questions for this book.
You are an inspiration to the entire field, and to me.
Thank you.*

FORWARD

There are physical therapists who are committed to the art and craft of physical therapy because of the lives they touch with their own hands, because of the opportunity to serve, because of the joy of making a difference one patient at at time. With contentment and balance in their lifestyles and finances, these therapists are not interested in salaries or talk of money in any way. For some, because their love of the profession is so great, discussion of income within the scope of PT life is viewed negatively.

There are physical therapists who are committed to the art and craft of physical therapy, who touch the lives of many with their own hands as they work for someone else, perhaps another therapist, perhaps a large company or a healthcare provider system, who feel like hamsters in a wheel, or a bees in a hive, working like mad to do another person's bidding. Substantial raises are a thing of the past. Life's expenses continue to rise, and with retirement savings not growing the promise of a golden future seems to be a fallacy. What would it be like if different choices had been made? What would it be like to own a PT business? These therapists, or those those who see this prophecy and want a different future, will benefit most from what is in this book.

There are physical therapists who are committed to the art and craft of physical therapy who touch countless lives not just with their own hands, who, by their talents, gather together therapists and employees together under one banner, as one company, and together make an impact far greater than one person ever could. These therapy business owners, innovators, and entrepreneurs, dedicated to the craft as they are, enjoy the rewards of a much higher income. Living with expanded means, they are afforded a different lifestyle than is common among therapists in the profession at large. These individuals will recognize the content of this book as their own story.

Three categories. Perhaps there are more. But for us, the question to consider is not which category describes us today, but which one will ten years from now.

—Chad Prince, February, 22 2016

INTRODUCTION

How much do physical therapists really make?
Are you in college and considering going into physical therapy?
Are you a PT already and curious about what others earn?

Have you hit the ceiling in your job and want to know what else is out there?

I asked myself those questions at one point or another in my career. Most therapists do.

The questions I wish I would have asked early in my career are these: Is the ladder that I'm climbing leaned against the right wall? Is the path I'm on going to give me the result I want in twenty years?

Want to know how you can have *above average* income as a PT? Want to know how to raise the ceiling and earn more? Want to know how to minimize the risks of starting your own practice, or how to make money on the side, or how to get in the *fastlane?*

You're in the right place.

In this book, we'll discuss many of the details surrounding physical therapist salaries. We'll cover starting salaries for new grads, salary growth during the first ten years of practice, and hitting the ceiling as a seasoned therapist. We'll also discuss ways to raise this ceiling, and how to create the illustrious *passive income* with entrepreneurialism. Along the way, we'll talk with several therapists who have started their own highly successful businesses, or who are on their way to fastlane success now, and you'll be given several references for books and articles on entrepreneurialism that will give you plenty of fuel to keep your fire hot for a long time to come.

What gives me the street credit to write a book like this?

Seven years ago, after a decade as a PT, I left physical therapy and began working full-time in healthcare administration. Now I manage a multi-million dollar business and have gained great insight into financial trends within medicine. One of the components under my watch is the contractual relationship between the practice I work for and a physical therapy company that employs PTs all across the country. I've learned a lot about what drives PT salaries, how much money therapy businesses really make and how much of that goes to their investors, how the financial climate affects therapist income levels, and ways PTs can raise their income. I've seen firsthand the effect of referrals drying up, and the cash flow created by a strong referral source. I've met several therapists like me who have left the field. I've met therapists who started their own companies, some that grew to the largest of their kind in the nation. I've talked with several who have found ways to expand their reach as a therapist, and who enjoy greater financial freedom while still treating patients on a daily basis.

Two concepts changed everything for me—"trading time for dollars," and **fastlane**. They inspired me to invent and bring to market new physical therapy products, the first of which is the UELadder, and to write this book.

Let me ask you again, do you want to know how you can have *above average* income as a PT?

Your answer might be, "No, I'm doing just fine, thank you very much." That's the case for plenty of therapists. I completely respect that.

But if you're on the fence, then let me give you a nudge. The last twenty years have not been very friendly to investors in the stock market. Unless you work for the state or federal government, you aren't going to have a pension for retirement. Everyone should be saving, but it's not easy with the rising costs of living. If earning more money meant saving more for your family, for your kids' college, for retirement, wouldn't that be worth it?

We *really* feel it the first year we get a nice raise. We get used to having more money. We adjust our lifestyles to this new income level, and we get comfortable. A five thousand dollar raise feels like a lot in the first year, but we forget it after three years. Still, that money has been coming in, and during those three years it was not just five thousand dollars, but fifteen thousand! After ten years that grows to fifty thousand!

If you let years pass by without trying to increase your income, then you're leaving money on the table, and for every year that passes that number gets higher and higher. You don't want to make that choice, do you?

You don't want to wake up in ten or twenty years and realize the ladder you've been climbing is leaned against the wrong wall, do you?

I didn't think so.

The book you need is in your hands. Let's get started.

INITIAL EVALUATION

SUBJECTIVE: Reader presents today with some interest in the topic covered by this book, and expresses hope that some path might be illuminated in such a way that he/she can take advantage of the information. Reader displays expressions of pain at the mention of income ceilings, but then takes on a guarded posture—arms folded across the chest and one hand over the sternum—while discussing the implications of increased salaries.

OBJECTIVE: Reader is informed that this book is part self-actualization and motivational coaching, part objective analysis of the current state of salaries within the physical therapy profession, and part assessment of career strategies, business opportunities, and entrepreneurial efforts that can be pursued with varying outcomes. Reader acknowledges this and consents to move ahead with Part 1: Loading Your Toolbox. After reading this and Part 2: The State of PT Salaries Today (which might not be necessary except for students or those new to the field), the reader has the choice of moving on to Part 3: The First Decade, or skipping ahead to Part 4: Raising the Ceiling. The reader is told that the Initial Evaluation, Re-certification, and Discharge sections are required in order to achieve the best outcome.

Links to external sources are included within this book, and the reader is encouraged to bookmark these for future follow-up. Additional materials that complement this book are also available at www.UELadder.com/pages/bonus-materials.

ASSESSMENT: The reader presents today with knowledge of physical therapy being a profession that has many strengths; that providing care to those in need is tremendously rewarding;

that PT is a noble career path, one that can be a launching pad for growth into many different fields of interests or business pursuits. Still, like so many therapists in the field today, the reader would like to learn more about physical therapy salaries, how to avoid income ceilings, and ways to maximize income. Skilled education is indicated that will progress toward the following goals:

1. Reader will read Part 1: Loading Your Toolbox within two days and complete assignments within a week in order to incorporate new daily routines into their life and to best achieve their personal vision.

2. Reader will print and sign the PTC&SG 30-Day Challenge and post it on their wall to remind themselves of their commitment.

3. Reader will connect with a colleague within one week of beginning this book and tell him or her about it so that they can begin a journey to professional growth together.

4. Reader will also connect with the Physical Therapy Business and Entrepreneur Accelerator (PTB&EA) Community and find like-minded colleagues and an environment of sharing all related to physical therapy salaries.

5. Reader will complete this book within a month, complete the 30-day challenge, then report ideas and progress to the PTB&EA Community.

PLAN: Reader will proceed through the pages of this book and discover ten interviews with physical therapy business leaders and entrepreneurs, condensed wisdom from multiple business authorities on strategy and business design, and an objective assessment of the current state of physical therapy salaries. Reader will find the most benefit by networking with like-minded professionals while reading this book and afterwards when incorporating these ideas into his or her professional life and career.

Part 1

Fill Your Toolbox

Chapter 1

Find Your Why

"He who has a why to live can bear almost any how."
Friedrich Nietzsche

Why write a book about PT Salaries?

You could have picked up this book for several reasons. Maybe you're curious. I hope not out of contempt, but I know that is a possibility. Maybe you're curious about PT incomes in general. Maybe you have pain in your current situation and you want to know if there is a way out of it—not every therapist loves his or her job, after all.

The idea of making more money is universally appealing, though being motivated only by money is usually seen as selfishness. Everyone could use some extra cash, but those who have ambition to amass great wealth are often shunned. This is widely accepted in society, and within physical therapy, a profession of service workers, the same holds true.

Let's listen to the words of several of the entrepreneurs interviewed later in this book as they talk about "why."

"If the only reason you're doing what you're doing is to make money, then maybe that's not the right reason. If you're only doing it for the money, then people are going to see right through that. I mean, you're not gonna get any referrals, I can tell you that." —Karen Litzy, DPT, of The Healthy, Wealthy & Smart Podcast

"First of all, I feel like success should never be defined in financial terms. I think that is one of the last definitions of success." —Tom Pennington, PT, CEO of Physicians Rehab Services

"I firmly believe that doing things solely to make more money will not lead to success." —Heidi Jannenga, DPT, President of WebPT

"Starting a business with only a monetary goal in mind is probably not a great idea." — Eric Gartner, PT, Founder of SimpleSet.net

What reasons are there for discussing PT salaries if successful entrepreneurs within the therapy world don't think it is a worthy goal? Pay closer attention to what they said: "If the *only* reason..." "Starting a business with *only* a monetary goal..." "...doing things *solely* to make more money..."

There are many reasons to strive for higher performance, and earning more is one of them, but *only* desiring more money is not healthy. As a component of a larger vision or purpose, wanting to earn more can be a noble goal. Clearly defining our personal mission is an exercise that everyone should undertake, both for the motivation it will give us in the present and for the direction it can give us in times of crisis.

Fourteen Reasons Why a PT Might Seek Higher Income

- Everyone can identify with the desire to have more spending money. Yes, this could be selfish, but maybe it's because you want to buy things for someone you love, or you want to spend the money taking your kids on vacation. Is this a bad thing?

- You want higher income so you can better save for retirement, or to pay off your student loans, or to save for your kids' college, or to pay for your daughter's wedding, or for ...

- Having more money to elevate your lifestyle could be viewed as thin and weak motivation, but it could be that you see a higher level lifestyle as proof that you have escaped from a difficult situation in your past.

- If you are frustrated by the current management at your job and feel the low ceiling in your department, then you may be motivated to move beyond that situation and prove to your current employer that they did not see your talent.

- You might simply want to be your own boss. You might want to hire other employees and be their boss, too.

- You think you're the best and want to prove it in the community with your own business.

- You have a vision for helping more people than just what you can do with your hands and your skills. This vision could be even bigger than what you can do with your team's hands and skills.

- You want to show that you can navigate the sea of healthcare change and continue to excel at PT and provide jobs for your team in the process.

- You want to create a business of value that you can sell later in life that will provide for you and your family in retirement.

- You want to make a difference in the therapy world at large, teaching other therapists your specialized skills.

- You want to reshape the therapy world at large, becoming a trendsetter and a movement starter within the profession. You want your name to be mentioned alongside of McKenzie and Maitland.

- You want your voice, and your unique talents and experiences blended with physical therapy, to be heard.

- You desire to have a different form of income that provides freedom from a nine-to-five job in order to spend more time with your family without sacrificing your lifestyle or savings.

- You desire to have a different form of income that provides freedom to pursue different paths like writing, missionary work, teaching, or speaking.

There are many noble "why's" when considering what motivates PT's to seek higher income. I've listed fourteen, but surely there are thousands. No doubt, only wanting more money is not a good reason to read this book, but even if a person has this singular motivation, it is almost impossible to achieve wealth in physical therapy without providing a lot of service to a lot of people. If "good people do bad things," isn't it also true that "bad people do good things?" It happens.

I want to challenge you to invest time in discovering your personal "why." Dig deep. Incorporate everything in your life, including your present life and your future children or grandchildren, your retirement, your home, your vacations, your contributions professionally, your social life, your spiritual life, your legacy. What do you want your life to mean? Decide. Write it down. Sure, it can change and evolve over time, and you should expect that this will happen. Still, distilling your passions into a vision can give you great clarity for evaluating the material and opportunities presented in this book.

Margie Warrell, a contributor to Forbes.com, wrote a post entitled: "Do You Know Your "Why?" 4 Questions To Find Your Purpose." Her four questions are:

- What makes you come alive?

- What are your innate strengths?

- Where do you add the greatest value?

- How will you measure your life?

Answering these questions is a great place to start on your road to self-discovery. In addition, Stephen Covey's book, *The 8th Habit: From Effectiveness to Greatness*, is all about finding your own "voice," which is essentially your "why."

"Why" write about PT Salaries? The bigger our "why," the bigger our impact, and the bigger our salaries will be.

Chapter 2

Build an Affirmation Statement

> *"It's about becoming the person who is worthy of achieving your goals."* —Hal Elrod

If you're reading this book hoping to gain some insights in how you can raise your income, then the first place to start is working on yourself. You will need to turn yourself into a person who deserves to earn more. To do that, you will need to build upon your clinical training with some business understanding.

The place to start this journey is with a self-assessment.

Here are a few questions to consider:

1. How well do you understand the forces that determine therapist salary levels?
2. How much do you understand about business? Do you have any business experience?
3. Are you a natural leader? Are there people who follow you?
4. Do you have passion to work hard, harder than anyone else, for a long time even if there is no return on your investment of energy?

5. Do you want to be the best in your field?
6. Do you look for ways to connect with other leaders in the profession?
7. Have you ever sold anything?
8. Are you proficient at basic computer skills? Do you have advanced computer experience?
9. Do you have any money set aside for savings?
10. Are you in a committed relationship with a person who supports your lifestyle with additional income?
11. Does this person share your vision for growing your career?
12. Are you afraid of losing a good thing?
13. Do you want to take action, but don't know what to do? Are you looking for an opportunity?
14. Do you have an idea of what the first six months of expenses in a business will be?
15. What are your thoughts on small business loans?
16. Do you have a mentor who can guide you through the process of starting and growing a business?
17. Do you have partners with skills that are different than your own who can help guide you through the difficult challenges within the business?
18. Do you understand the long-term path where your business idea leads?
19. Do you understand how taxes work for a business owner, including the advantages and disadvantages of different business structures?
20. Have you thought about hiring staff? What criteria will you use to filter out the right people? How do you budget for their salaries?
21. What will you do when you don't have enough cash to meet payroll?

22. Do you know the difference between marketing and branding?
23. Do you think having a website is enough?
24. Are you ready to work in an administrative role as well as being a clinician— for no more pay—for a long time?
25. Do you know anything about billing, or do you have a strong connection with a biller?
26. Do you have a five-year business plan to estimate expenses?
27. Do you have a strength that gives you an unfair advantage, that will set you apart in the marketplace from other therapy businesses?
28. Do you have connections with referral sources, or a method of gaining and growing your business?
29. Are you geographically located in an area that is ideal for your strengths?
30. Have you ever heard of Sales and Use Tax?

If I've overwhelmed you, that's okay. You don't have to be an expert on all of these topics before going forward in your career. You don't have to get it perfectly right on day one in order to hit an acquisition target 25 years in the future. That being said, the more you understand, the better choices you will be able to make.

The purpose of this exercise is not to shatter your confidence but to illustrate where you are at the moment. As therapists, we all take measurements of post-op total knee replacement patients at the initial evaluation. Our patients invariably ask, "Was that good?"

Sure, it would be better if a patient has one hundred and twenty degrees of flexion, and, yes, it is not great if they only have seventy-five, but we all tell the patient the same thing: initial measurements are not good or bad, they are just a starting point. What matters the most are the measurements at discharge! If you don't have a lot of business savvy or know-how right now, that is okay. Have confidence in yourself. You are already a PT, or you are well on your way to becoming one. This, by itself, is no small feat.

When we are outside of our comfort zone, we often succumb to FEAR. FEAR stands for False Evidence Appearing Real, and it can stop almost anyone in their tracks. In order to combat fear, you have to have the right kind of confidence. Being cocky, as we all know, is really just trying to hide self-doubt. True confidence doesn't act like a know-it-all, but rather works to find answers to questions, and applies those answers to build success.

As a therapist, this is a skill you already have. You are a clinically trained problem-solver.

Business is often much less complex than clinical practice, but it can be scarier because the stakes are higher. Still, I fully believe therapists can rapidly gain proficiency in business skills by adopting a few daily habits and by thinking of themselves as already being successful business leaders.

What is an affirmation?

Popular psychology books and many business philosophy experts teach about the power of human thought and self-talk. We all understand that thinking negatively will erode confidence, and we see the benefits of thinking positively. Replacing "I'm no good" with "I'm just fine – I'm me" has been a mantra for so many movements. Having a daily affirmation is taking this a step further.

A daily affirmation is the process of choosing who you need to be in order to accomplish everything you want, and then telling yourself you are already that person. "I AM THE GREATEST!" Muhammad Ali affirmed these words over and over again until he *was* the greatest.

Some affirmations are ridiculous. Hal Elrod, bestselling author of *The Miracle Morning*, gives these examples:

I am a millionaire. *No, you're not.*

I have 7 percent body fat. *No, you don't.*

I have achieved all off my goals this year. *Nope. Sorry, you haven't.*

Hal goes on to give four simple steps for creating affirmations that work:
1. Build it around the result you are committed to and why.
2. Describe necessary actions you are committed to taking and when.
3. Recite your affirmations every morning.
4. Constantly update and evolve your affirmations.

Today, challenge yourself to craft a personalized affirmation statement about who you want to become. Do you want higher income as a physical therapist? Then see yourself as a person who deserves to be paid more because of the financial value you bring to the marketplace.

Here is a sample affirmation:

I am (or am going to be) a physical therapist. This is a great accomplishment in and of itself, and is proof that I can learn and master a huge body of knowledge of complex and detailed material. I certainly didn't know it all on the first day of class, but each day I worked to learn more and more. If I want to avoid income ceilings as a PT, I'm going to have to learn how to position myself for opportunities and then be ready to take them. Every day, I will learn something that will make me a more skilled therapist, a stronger leader, a business-minded professional, a confident risk-evaluator, and a calculated risk-taker. Lots of other therapists in the world have avoided income ceilings, and they are no smarter than I am. I can do it too, but it won't happen by itself. I am learning every day. I am pushing myself every day. I am growing every day. I have been and will be challenged. I may fail but I will get back up. I am and will be successful.

I challenge you to craft your own affirmation statement, one that blends your skills and talents with your goals and desires to create a vision of who you want to be. Start working on it today!

"Let today be the day you give up who you've been for who you can become." —Hal Elrod

Chapter 3

Create Daily Routines

To become a better version of yourself, one that deserves to perform at a higher level and earn higher income as a result, you will have to create some new routines.

My suggestion is for you to make time every day to go through the following steps. Let's call it your Physical Therapy Career & Salary Guide checklist, and we'll use the initials PTCSG to help you remember the steps:

- Put your affirmations & visions in your head and heart.
- Track your progress with journaling.
- Challenge your status quo.
- Share your journey with a friend and colleague.
- Grow: read, listen, and watch to develop new skills.

Step One is to *put your affirmations and visions into your head and heart*. You can do this by saying them aloud. Hear yourself saying them. There's a lot of power to help overcome fear in hearing your own voice saying that you are strong and smart and capable of achieving great things. Your "why" will be a compass to you, and repeating it will remind you of your priorities and your purpose. Life is full of distractions and tangents, so knowing "why" can really keep you on track.

Step Two is to *track your progress with journaling*. There are a lot of tools available on the market for this. *The Freedom Journal* and *The Five-Minute Journal* are two that are designed for achievers, but you can get great value in recording your progress in a book with blank pages or even in a simple word processing document. Keep a record of the things you learn and the places you learn them. It is great to be able to reference articles, blogs, books, and course material from years back.

Step Three is to *challenge your status quo*. What are you doing about your health and fitness? How are you managing your money? How is your spiritual life? How much time do you spend on meaningless entertainment? How well is your future or your family's future protected if something were to happen to your ability to work? Explore these areas of life. Growth in one area can stimulate development and habit formation in others.

Look for evidence of abundance. It's amazing what we can see when we look for something specific. Look for people who have what you desire, whether it's fitness, money, solid relationships, deep spirituality, security, or opportunity. Study their habits, their routines. Learn how they got to where they are. Challenge yourself to move from where you are today to where you want to be. This is a long journey, but it begins by getting yourself out of your own status quo.

Step Four is to *share your journey with a friend and colleague.* Hopefully this person will take the journey with you. Share your strengths, your weaknesses, and what you learn along the way. Learn from each other. The more you talk about it, the more likely you will grow into the person you want to be.

Maybe you don't have close colleagues who are interested in developing themselves professionally. Connect with us through the [Physical Therapy Business & Entrepreneur Accelerator Facebook Community](http://www.facebook.com/groups/PTBizAccelerator/). There you will find like-minded therapists who are striving for some of the same goals as you.

http://www.facebook.com/groups/PTBizAccelerator/

Step Five is to *Grow. Read, listen, and watch in order to develop new skills.* It's not enough just to say "read." For me, I don't have time to sit and read, but I love to listen. I wear my Bluetooth headphones three or four hours every day, listening to books from Audible and Overdrive, podcasts, and pdfs read by an app called Voice Dream. The amount of information available on almost every business topic is astounding. You can't learn everything you need to know in a month or even a year. Start reading and learning something that will help you grow every day.

Add to this list some of your own routines, but it will be important to make these the core of your new daily habits.

"We are what we repeatedly do. Excellence, then, is not an act, but a habit." —Aristotle

Chapter 4

30-Day Challenge

I, _____, hereby challenge myself to make time every day to:

- Put my affirmations & visions in my head and heart.
- Track my progress with journaling.
- Challenge my status quo.
- Share my journey with a friend and colleague.
- Grow: Read, listen, and watch so that I can develop new skills.

I will make a note of my commitment to this in my daily journal, I will share it with my friends and colleague, and I will tell others about my progress.

_____ _____
Signature   Date

Part 2

The State of PT Salaries Today

Chapter 5

How Much Do PTs Make?

When it comes to writing notes and documentation, if it's possible to have a favorite part, mine is the objective section of a note. I love that you can jump from one finding to another without connecting the dots. Yes, there could be some flow. For example, I could record range of motion, then strength measurements, then special tests. But within each section I could jump around, first giving range of motion at the ankle, then at the hip, then strength at the knee. While a bit disjointed, we all know that for documentation purposes this is just fine. This next section is a bit that way. We'll cover salaries at a high level, look at the pros of the physical therapy profession, explore the healthcare climate to see its effect on PT, discuss several business structures within the physical therapy profession, and finally examine some of the negative parts of life as a physical therapist. Some of this will be elementary and won't mean much to you. Other parts could be enlightening. My goal is to paint the big picture of the profession—as I see it, of course—including strengths and weaknesses, to get us on the same page as we look at opportunities in upcoming sections.

Let's get started.

How much do PTs make?

At present, a Google search of physical therapist salaries returns an average salary of $80,000. This really doesn't tell us a lot, does it?

PayScale.com gives a more conservative estimate of $67,000. This website also says that the highest paying fields within physical therapy are home health, long-term care, and geriatrics. I don't disagree with this statement, but it still doesn't give us a very full picture.

Salary.com gives a range between $73,500 and $86,500 for physical therapist salaries. It also gives a graph of a bell shaped curve with 10% of salaries below $68,000, 25% below $73,500, a mid-range of $80,000, 75% below $86,600, and 90% below $93,000. This is the most complete information that we have so far. You can purchase a full report from this website that breaks down salary information even further, considering your state and other specific details that could change the data.

Salary information that is publicly available vs. reality

Imagine cheerleaders and pompoms and lots of jumping up and down. This was quite a scene for our PT school class but one day out of the blue two students burst into the classroom dressed as the Spartan cheerleaders from *Saturday Night Live*. Their cheer went like this:

"It depends
It, it depends
I say it— you say depends

It
Depends
It
Depends"

Everyone went crazy laughing and clapping because this phrase was a favorite among our professors. They told us it would shape our decisions every day as physical therapists. The phrase is true in practice, and it's true for physical therapist salaries.

Okay, so "it depends." What does that mean?

Just as in real estate, the three most important factors for physical therapist salaries are as follows:

Location
Location
Location

There is more to it than this, but it really makes a difference where you are trying to practice. Some states pay more for physical therapists because the Medicare Fee Schedule is higher. Within each state there are urban and rural areas, and contrary to what you might think, rural areas pay the most. This is because rural areas are not as desirable as urban areas. When you take into consideration the lower cost of living in rural areas, therapists who are willing to venture into the sticks to work really have opportunities for higher incomes. Don't be surprised if someone in your class who goes to work in Roanoke, Alabama has a higher starting salary than someone who goes to work in Roanoke, Virginia.

Ben Fung has some very good information available on the 2015 physical therapy job market at this site: http://updocmedia.com/2015-pt-job-market-outlook-v2/. Another great resource available from WebPT is titled Four Things You Need to Know About PT Salary: https://www.webpt.com/blog/post/four-things-you-need-know-about-pt-salary. Keep in mind that tabular data changes constantly and varies within each state.

I asked Lee Cummings, a regional manager for Integrity Rehab Group, what factors influenced him to offer a new grad top pay. Here's his answer:

"The determining factor is location and market. In places like Tulsa, Oklahoma, PTs are easy to come by and therefore easier to hire at the lower end of the scale. However, Chickasha, Oklahoma is a very difficult place to find and recruit a therapist, and so at times we have to go higher on the scale to get someone in."

As we have already discussed, there are areas within physical therapist practice that pay more. The burning question that we need to answer is: Why?

Physical therapist salaries are directly connected to the revenue generated by the therapist, generally 30-60% of that revenue. No matter what setting, if the business has a structure or a payment source or payer mix that pays well, PTs can expect to be paid a higher amount. If there is lower payment, therapists will be paid less.

In home health, therapists work one-on-one with patients in their homes. The care is often basic because the type of care patients need at this point in their recovery process is basic, and because the equipment you can provide is limited to what you can take with you to the visit. Still, home health is paid well for this service, and PT salaries in this setting are at the top of the spectrum. Comparing home health to outpatient pediatric therapy, where a high percentage of patients require one-on-one therapy but a lower level of revenue is generated, it follows that therapists in this setting have salaries at the lower end of the spectrum.

The same scenario applies to outpatient physical therapy. Clinics where therapists regularly see two patients an hour will generate more revenue than clinics that only see one patient per hour. The more revenue that is generated, the higher salaries should be. Large corporations with large clinics and many layers of corporate overhead to maintain will have to pay therapists a lower percentage of overall revenue than a smaller practice with tightly controlled overhead.

For more information about this, check out Greg Todd's YouTube video entitled *Let's Talk Physical Therapist Salaries,* (https://www.youtube.com/watch?v=JxNujKZxPn4). Take a minute and check this video out — it's great!

Home health has probably the highest pay, but this may not be the best location for a new grad PT. Working alone in a patient's home has risks. If something goes wrong you won't have back-up help from other therapists. That's not to say new grads can't go to work in the highest paying field right out of school, but it is a consideration that in the early phases of your career you may want other therapists close by for support.

Long-term care is another high paying area of physical therapy. Generally in this setting there are other therapists around, though in rural settings these may be PTAs, OTs, COTAs, or SLPs. I learned as much from experienced PTAs as I did other PTs.

Geriatrics is a higher paying field because most patients have Medicare, which reimburses well in skilled nursing facilities and in home health. Contrast this with pediatrics, in which many patients who need services either have private insurance, state insurance (Medicaid), or no insurance. Pediatrics typically requires one-on-one care. Less revenue is generated, so pediatric therapists don't make as much. Sometimes jobs in pediatrics are associated with hospitals, and sometimes they are associated with school systems. Working directly for a school system may have lower pay but it also might have better benefits and more time off (all school holidays). Contracting with a school system is a different matter altogether, and we'll talk about this later.

Outpatient physical therapy is being affected by high deductible insurance plans. For forward-thinking clinics, this is an advantage. For others, it is a major hurdle. Physical therapy services, generally, are applied to a patient's deductible. All charges will have to be paid for out-of-pocket until the deductible is met. With deductibles commonly three thousand dollars and above, this can mean that a patient has to pay for an entire PT episode themselves. This may decrease utilization of physical therapy and decrease clinic revenue.

I spoke with a friend and colleague who manages a large territory. He told me that the company he works for tries to hire new grad therapists in the $60,000 - $65,000 range. However, if revenues begin to fall for this section of the market then we can expect salaries to decrease overtime in this area, as well.

This brings us to a very important point regarding salaries: timing.

At my first job I worked with two therapists who graduated from the same PT program I did, but two years before me. They received multiple job offers, high salaries, and $10,000 sign-on bonuses. During the next two years while I was in physical therapy school, there was national legislation passed that reshaped long-term care physical therapy. The market was flooded with physical therapists and salaries plummeted. When my class met for the last time for graduation, only five of us (out of fifty) had jobs. Sign-on bonuses? Forget about it. Overall, my class was offered salaries almost $20,000 a year less than therapists who graduated two years earlier.

There's not a lot that you can do to protect yourself against changes in the national marketplace for physical therapists. Fortunately, within two to three years after I graduated the job market recovered and opportunities for therapists to get jobs quickly returned. Unfortunately, the high sign-on bonuses for new grads did not return. Now, almost twenty years later, sign-on bonuses are back, but this is more related to less desirable parts of the country. Want to work in an upscale metro area? Don't expect a sign-on bonus. Are you willing to go to rural Louisiana or Mississippi? You might see a nice sign-on bonus, but you might have to work there two to three years to get forgiveness.

No matter where you work, try to learn how much revenue therapists generate in the business. Employers may not want to share exact numbers, but you can do research and get a feel for revenue based on caseload volume. As you gain confidence and experience, the way to leverage this information to gain higher pay is to show that you can see higher volumes.

Suggestions for getting a top salary at your first job

1. Do a great job in clinical training so you have positive references, and perhaps one of your clinical sites will hire you.

2. Interview at more than one place. Hopefully you'll get more than one offer. Then you can take your pick or even counteroffer to get a higher salary.

3. Recommendation: *Salary Tutor* by Jim Hopkinson

****

Reminder — Daily routines? Do you have them set yet? A great book on this is *Automate Your Routines Guarantee Your Results* by Kathryn Jones

http://amzn.to/1TR2vjJ

****

Chapter 6

The Pros of Physical Therapy

Next, let's look at all the positives that are part of a career in physical therapy. There's a reason why so many people are on the waiting list to get into PT school every year...

1. **Rewarding career using specialized knowledge to help people in significant ways.** Physical therapy is a wonderful profession. It is very fulfilling to be able to have a significant impact on the lives of others. The happiest times of my career I worked in a setting where I could provide care to patients in short-term rehab who really made fast progress and who had a huge appreciation for my team of therapists, and I also worked in an outpatient clinic within the same business, which met my needs for high-level interventions. There was enough variety to keep me satisfied, and I truly felt I was having an impact with the patients we saw and in the community.

2. **Job opportunities.** It is an incredible advantage to know that, regardless of where you live, you can find work. Anywhere there are people there will be a need for physical therapy. Because many jobs are hard to fill, there are even opportunities for traveling PTs with short-term assignments all over the country.

3. **Several career paths within the profession**. Physical therapists take care of patients in all phases of life, literally from the cradle to the grave. There is specialization within the field, and jobs that focus just on specific areas of practice. The major categories of the profession are Pediatrics, Acute Care, Inpatient Rehabilitation at acute rehabilitation hospitals, Short-Term Rehabilitation and Long-Term Care in skilled nursing facilities, Home Health, Outpatient, and Sports Enhancement. Many jobs and businesses are focused just on one area of specialization. Some have a general focus and help patients who have a variety of problems, even allowing therapists to work in two or more distinct areas of practice at the same time. While each of these subsets has its own unique pros and cons, each appealing to therapists in different ways, the good thing is there isn't so much specialization that therapists can't make a complete career move. I've seen many therapists flip-flop between home health and outpatient therapy. One of the best pieces of advice I ever received was that my first job be in a setting where several types of physical therapy were provided. I worked at a hospital, and got to experience wound care, acute care, outpatient therapy, and home health, all with one employer. From there I was confident to move into a job that involved both outpatient and short-term rehab.

4. **Comfortable living**. Yes, the rewards of PT are great in and of themselves. Yes, job opportunities are abundant and the opportunity to make more money is available if a person wants it. General PT salaries provide a comfortable living. My wife was a stay-at-home mom for nine years and we made it just fine on my PT income. Of course, we had to be careful with our money, but that is required at most salary levels.

5. **Steady salary increases in first ten years of practicing.** It's absolutely thrilling to see your income increase rapidly. You get used to it. You think that it's going to continue to go up. All students start out a good deal lower than the average, so there is a lot of room to have increases at the beginning of a PT career.

6. **Opportunities for advancement without relocating.** Even in the smallest towns there are probably a few different types of physical therapy being provided. Most companies will be willing to hire a physical therapist with some experience to take on the management of their rehabilitation department. It might not be the career direction you thought you would take in PT school, but increasing responsibility increases salary.

7. **Greater opportunities for advancement with relocation.** Physical therapy companies can be huge. The larger the company, the more regional managers they will need. If a PT gains experience in management then doors can open all over the country. Increasing responsibility brings increased salaries and increased bonus opportunities, but it can also bring extensive travel.

8. **Prestige.** Physical therapists are highly regarded and highly sought after.

9. **PRN work.** "PRN" stands for "as needed." Nursing homes, schools, and home health agencies need extra help all the time. A good way to make extra money is to spend a few hours each month doing PRN work. Outpatient clinics need coverage from time to time when therapists are on vacation or on maternity leave. If you can give up benefits and consistent income, therapists who work PRN make high hourly rates and have lots of flexibility.

10. **Provide education.** There is the option to further your own education and teach in a university, as a clinical instructor of students, as a provider of continuing education, or through websites and online communities. Did I mention there are lots of opportunities?

11. **Option to perform research.** This is largely associated with university settings.

12. **Huge marketplace for entrepreneurial developments.** (Did the word "entrepreneur" get your attention? More on this later ...)

****

***Reminder** — [The Physical Therapy Business & Entrepreneur Accelerator Community](http://www.facebook.com/groups/PTBizAccelerator/) is a great place to interact with other therapists about any questions you have about this book.*
    http://www.facebook.com/groups/PTBizAccelerator/
****

Chapter 7

Health Care Challenges

President John F. Kennedy said, "A rising tide lifts all boats." Professions within the healthcare field are affected positively and negatively by global forces on industry. This certainly applies to physical therapy.

1. In the past 25 years (and perhaps even before), **insurance companies have had the upper hand in the medical world at large**. Medicare is the driving force behind decreasing reimbursement. When Medicare lowers their fee schedule, all of the private insurances do the same. This means that PTs have no control over how much we will be paid for the services we give. We can charge whatever we want to charge for the work we do, but we will only be paid what the insurance company says is allowable. In today's world, less and less is allowable. This creates an unfortunate business environment where the same amount of work performed last year will bring a business less money this year. Providers have to seek patient populations, which have problems that have high reimbursement. Patients without insurance are often considered undesirables.

2. **High deductible insurance plans make it hard for a lot of patients to pay for the care they need**. In the past three years, there has been a big shift for patients to have to pay more of their bill and for providers to have to collect that money from the patient. This means that in addition to decreased reimbursement from the insurance company, more of the payment that we will receive as providers and that we need to stay in business will come directly from the patient. Unfortunately, many times when a patient needs care they are not prepared financially to pay for the care they need. Providers are left with the ethical dilemma of whether or not to render services to someone who might not be able to pay. This was much less of an issue when the patient portion was 5–10% of the total amount expected to be collected. With high deductible plans, this amount is sometimes 50–100% of the total amount to be collected. Most private insurance plans require the deductible to be met fully before they will cover physical therapy. With a high deductible plan this might mean that every physical therapy visit will have to be paid out of the patient's pocket. At $100 per visit this adds up quickly and can be a burden that patients cannot bear. So, they don't bear it, and many choose not to get physical therapy at all.

3. **The cost of doing business continues to rise with inflation**. Along with decreased reimbursement, there have been increases in the cost of providing employees insurance. There are many other increases in business costs, as well. The healthcare industry is facing the unfortunate convergence of decreasing reimbursement and increasing costs. Basically, the profit in healthcare is being squeezed.

4. Due to the pressures on healthcare at large, pressures that certainly affect PT, **it is becoming more and more difficult for independent practitioners to survive**.

This is true of physicians and physical therapists alike. Large corporations are growing because they can manage providers at a lower overall cost of doing business due to economies of scale. The infrastructure to manage five therapy outpatient clinics is not that much different than what is needed to manage 50 clinics. This is true for almost any setting within healthcare. Physicians are selling their practices to hospitals or to large groups for management. Long-term care facilities are selling to national chains.

5. **A landscape dominated by large corporations results in the leveling of salaries and benefits, which will help some and hurt others**. Large corporations create ladders that can be climbed. This provides opportunities for advancement, but it also creates well-defined roles for therapists. Generally, corporations do not want their staff to deviate from these roles. Therapists are not asked to create programs; they are told which programs to use that are created by the corporate office. Therapists are to treat patients, and corporate will take care of the rest.

6. **The practice of medicine is driven by physicians**. Physical therapists are considered mid-level providers similar to pharmacists and nurse practitioners. In a few states, therapists are able to treat patients on their own without a physician referral, but even there, reimbursement can be limited without a physician directing care. This means that physician referrals are critical to the success of any PT business. No matter how successful a practice has been in the past, if physician referrals dry up the practice can have significant financial problems. This is less relevant to long-term care and more relevant to outpatient physical therapy businesses, but the risk is still there.

7. **A landscape dominated by large, equity-backed companies and physician-owned clinics will take the profit out of PT for the investors, limiting salary opportunity for PTs.** How much profit? As much as 40% of total revenue. Therapists may be asked to see a high volume of patients, decreasing the amount of interaction they can have with each patient and reducing the fulfillment that can be felt from providing care, all so the profit lost from decreasing reimbursement and increasing overhead can be recovered for investors. Many therapists feel like highly educated worker bees in hives they do not own with queens they do not know.

8. **Time for money.** Healthcare, in almost every scenario, requires direct interaction with patients. There is very little opportunity for passive income. More on this later.

9. **Healthcare providers at large are not in control of their own destiny** because of declining reimbursement and national legislation that affects reimbursement. More on this later, as well.

Chapter 8

Physical Therapy Business Models

Get ready — we're about to talk chocolate!

Just as there are several areas of physical therapy practice, there are several business structures within the healthcare field and within physical therapy. Before we dive into the different structures, let's talk for a minute about basic business principles in terms that we all can enjoy: candy bars.

If you're selling candy bars, you need customers who will pay you, a storefront of some type, a means of attracting customers to your store, and candy bars themselves. You'll sell all day long and at the end of the day add up your money. This is called "gross sales." But gross sales is not the profit you made. No, the candy bars, the advertising, and the store itself all have a cost. This is called "overhead." Your profit is gross sales minus overhead.

Profit = Income - Overhead

To make money you have to charge enough per candy bar that you can pay for all of your costs. An ideal business has high income and low overhead. Of course, if you buy more candy bars or advertise more, overhead will go up. If you move to a storefront with cheaper rent your overhead will go down. If you're not making enough money you can try to sell more candy bars (which might mean more advertising), you could raise your prices, or you could lower your overhead. These are the general tactics used to increase profit.

Healthcare business has the same basic components—overhead is made up of buildings and equipment and staff and advertising. Income comes from getting paid for providing services. Profit comes from subtracting overhead from income—*but under the hood, things get more complicated.*

Income comes as a result of providing services and being paid by insurance companies and patients. Here's one of the big differences between healthcare and our candy bar example: healthcare providers can charge whatever they want, but, as we have already discussed, they will only be paid the "allowed amount" based on the contract they have with each insurance company. (Insurance companies are businesses, too, and one way they lower their overhead is by negotiating low contract rates.) Guess what? Each insurance company has its own allowable amounts. Some are higher than others and some are low. Seeing a mix of patients with different types of insurance is the norm, and the ideal situation is to have a high percentage of patients with high insurance allowable amounts. This factor of profit is called "payer mix."

Think this is complicated? We're just scratching the surface.

If the ideal is to have a strong payer mix, then all providers should just make this stronger, right? Sometimes it's possible, with marketing and superior service. Sometimes it's not, because of the economic situation in the city or town where the provider works.

Income comes from payment from insurance companies AND from patients. Recently, high deductible insurance plans have been brought into prominence. As a result, "payer mix" is a little less important and the ability of the patient to pay becomes critical. When a procedure or service "applies to deductible," the patient has to pay for the procedure out of their own pocket up to the amount of their deductible before their insurance will pay anything. Could this make a difference in profit? A major difference.

There's one more major income component in healthcare: volume. Volume covers a multitude of sins. With it, providers can enjoy stable business and grow; without it, providers will scramble to cover their costs. In general, volume comes from the community surrounding a healthcare business. It's no different for therapists, but we have to remember that physician referrals are necessary in almost every situation. Physician relations, then, are key to keeping volumes high.

Profit = Income - Overhead

Let's not forget the other element in the profit equation: overhead. Overhead is made up of facilities, equipment, supplies, advertising and marketing, personnel and staff benefits, as well as management and corporate compliance efforts (this is ensuring the facility is in alignment with all regulations that govern delivery of care and billing for services). The larger the business, the more complex the overhead.

Many of these elements are essential in healthcare. A nice, updated facility is necessary so that patients and physicians will choose to use you (a key to volume), but it is not without cost. Wherever there is an abundance of volume, expect competition, which will require large advertising budgets. Healthcare services can't be delivered without staff, but the ideal is to have just the right amount of staff for the job and not too many.

Management and corporate compliance can be consolidated between multiple offices. A small team of administrative professionals can manage multiple healthcare facilities, saving costs for all of them. This allows a facility to lower its overhead, thus increasing profits.

Consolidation of management not only allows facilities lower overhead, but it also broadens the experience of the administrative professionals who manage multiple facilities. They are able to apply what is learned in one facility to another, thus speeding up the adaptation of all facilities to the constant changes in the healthcare field.

Let's take these principles and see how they apply to different physical therapy business models. Each business structure, from the simple to the complex, relies on profit to stay in business. Each one has advantages and disadvantages, both for the business at large and for physical therapists.

1. Large, multidiscipline businesses

Hospitals, skilled nursing facilities, and home health agencies provide many types of healthcare. Rehabilitation services are a component of this larger picture. No matter how big, the same business tenants apply: profit comes from income minus overhead. Income can be huge, but so can overhead. Immense marketing is required to keep volume up. Lowering overhead is essential, and department managers constantly have to justify the number of staff they have on payroll. Consolidation of senior management is common, and there is a large corporate world with many publicly traded companies that have operations in multiple locations.

Therapists who work in these environments can enjoy the ease of having volume provided for them, the relief of having their corporate compliance programs developed and monitored, and the security of knowing that multidisciplinary organizations have great chances of weathering the storms of healthcare. It can also be very rewarding to work in a multidiscipline team that is providing care for an individual patient.

The negatives for therapists in these settings include: limited independence from management oversight and the direction of the larger organization; having no voice to be heard by leaders of the organization; the feeling of being just "another cog in the wheel," or just a "worker bee;" and income potential determined by the organization, usually not by the hard work of the therapist.

2. Rehabilitation-only companies

There are businesses that focus only on rehabilitation: physical therapy, occupational therapy, and speech/language pathology. These can be contract companies that provide services to hospitals or nursing homes, or they can be Certified Outpatient Rehabilitation Facilities (CORF). Businesses of this type are very scalable, meaning corporate management can provide infrastructure to support facilities or contracts for services in many locations.

Typically, CORFs are more vulnerable to the ebb and flow of volume than hospital-based therapy departments. Corporate compliance programs can come from the corporate headquarters, but it is likely that local therapists will have to teach and monitor these programs. The reward of working with only PT, OT, and SLP is just as strong as working with nursing services and other disciplines, but therapists can enjoy greater leadership in the decision-making process with patients that do not require other disciplines.

Contract businesses for PT, OT, and SLP that provide services in hospitals and nursing homes will have work experiences for their employees that are much the same as those of large, multidiscipline facilities. The main difference is that these therapists have a different employer. Sometimes this gives therapists a greater voice within the company, but other times the customer organization treats them and their company as dispense commodities.

3. Physical therapy-only businesses

It is possible for PT-only businesses to provide contract therapy, usually as subcontractors to hospitals, nursing homes and home health agencies, but most PT-only businesses are in the outpatient therapy arena.

Outpatient physical therapy businesses can be made up of one clinic, or hundreds of clinics that stretch all across the country. They can have a general focus, or be niche-based. They can hire physical therapists, physical therapist assistants, and athletic trainers, or they may choose to hire only physical therapists. There are successful business examples out there for every business structure nuance, too.

It is common for therapists who have one successful clinic to open another clinic in a different location. Many small-chain businesses exist where one or more owners have 5-10 outpatient clinics. There are large-scale businesses with hundreds of clinics that have reached their size by acquisition of smaller clinics and by expansion. These can be publicly traded companies or have private equity backing.

All of the forces that affect any healthcare business affect outpatient physical therapy. Small, single clinic operations as well as national, 100+ clinic organizations have to comply with governmental regulations. They all are affected equally if reimbursement changes, and they all can be independently affected by the ebb and flow of volume and by the changes in their unique referral sources.

There is greater stability in the larger organizations, but there is also greater corporate involvement and direction. Therapists may appreciate the job security that a large corporation can provide and the insulation they give that protects against sudden change, but they may resent having to document and follow guidelines provided by the corporation.

Physician referrals make a huge difference in outpatient clinics. It is common for non-therapists to be owners of these companies, and their interests are bottom-line oriented. They want to see profits. To compensate for risk and to level out referrals, some physical therapists and rehab companies have partnered with physicians so that the referring physician owns part of the business. While controversial, this arrangement has been found to be legal in most states. It creates a very steady flow of referrals, which creates job stability for therapists.

Unfortunately for outpatient clinics that are not physician-owned, physicians can open their own outpatient physical therapy clinic and direct referrals to their clinic that were once going to established clinics. A physical therapist who has been in business for years and has established a solid business in the community can see a major decline in volume when a physician-owned clinic opens. The threat of a physician-owned clinic opening next door can limit an individual physical therapist from opening his or her own practice because the risk of referrals drying up is always prevalent.

4. The solo physical therapist.

Physical therapists can be the owners and operators of their own businesses. These can take on many forms. Contracting independently to provide services to other therapy businesses is one form, but when most people think about someone owning their own business, that thought is accompanied by visions of a storefront. In PT, that storefront would be an outpatient clinic with either a general or a specialized focus.

A business like this will have all the overhead components that a large business does, and enough volume will be needed to pay this overhead before any profit is realized.

One distinct factor is a huge difference maker, though: 100% physical therapist ownership. This factor has nothing to do with the pride of owning your own business; what is significant is that there are not investors or other owners to take the profit out of the business.

It is generally true that profit margins increase as volume increases, and solo physical therapists can have difficulty gaining and maintaining steady volume. And remember, if no one is working, no money is coming into the business—a vacation for a solo physical therapist is a week without pay.

Still, if there is a steady stream of patients and if overhead is low, a therapist can see fewer patients each day and still generate enough revenue to have the same living as someone working in a busy clinic with elaborate equipment and investors who take the profit.

****

Reminder — daily affirmations, remember those?
Yep, they're important! Go back and revisit that section if needed, but I can't stress enough how much this can help overcome fear and uncertainty!
****

Chapter 9

The Cons of Physical Therapy

Every profession has pros and cons. Every situation does, every person does, every book does. The things that make a profession good for one person may not be the same for another. The things that turn one person away from a career field may be the very things that draw another to the same path. That being said, most people will agree with my list of pros. The cons, however, will irritate some more than others.

1. **95-99% of PTs "trade time for money."** What does this mean? Any job where you have to work a set number of hours in a pay period in order to get paid is a job that trades time for money. That doesn't mean it won't have a high salary. There are lots of high-paying jobs that fall into this classification—take physicians, for example. In my work with physicians I have grown to appreciate that if they take a vacation the money stops flowing. As a physical therapist you will have paid time off, but you're only allowed so much. Physical therapy is not the type of career where you can make money passively. This is important because of the lifestyle limitations it will place on things like extended travel and retirement. It's also important

because the place where you trade your time is at the clinic, at the hospital, or in a patient's home. Want to work from your living room? That's probably not going to happen unless you're in management, and even then it probably will not be every day.

2. **It is easy to hit an income ceiling after ten years of practice.** Why? More on this later.

3. While there are still lots of job openings, **after ten years of practice it can be hard to find new opportunities that are exciting** without relocating or being willing to travel. Opportunities available to you could be with companies or therapists that you have already worked with and that you don't want work with again. You could also have experience with different areas of PT practice where you may not want to work again; for example, in home health or outpatient therapy. Basically, after ten years of practice you will know what you like and what you don't like, and there may not be job opportunities that pay more money in your area.

4. Physical therapists are "mid-level" providers. This means that we do not have autonomy and have to work under the direction of a physician. While therapists are experts in movement and have intensive education and training, this distinction applies a ceiling to the profession.

5. Physical therapy is part of the overall healthcare system. While this provides great security because there will always be a need for our services, it also means that if the industry as a whole undergoes a crisis, so will physical therapy.

6. Therapists who want to go into business on their own face two huge challenges: financial risk and competition. These two factors are significant enough that many therapists feel

that going into business on their own simply isn't an option.

7. The reward of taking care of people in need is enough to overcome all of this, right? Yes, and no. It's wonderful to help people. The trouble is, there are many forces surrounding patient care that can cause burnout. **The fulfillment that comes from helping people diminishes if you're burned out, especially after you have treated hundreds of knees, shoulders, etc**.

8. Even though physical therapy is a profession with an immense body of knowledge, **the daily practice of physical therapy can become very routine**. Yes, outpatient clinics have lots of exercise equipment, but as a physical therapist you will be in that setting day in and day out. Home health therapists are able to move around a lot, but the therapy they provide is limited to equipment that a patient has in their home or that the therapist can bring with them. It's common for long-term care therapists to travel from one facility to another, but even if you are working with three or four facilities this too can become mundane. Just as in any profession, the setting becomes less important over time, and if we do the same thing over and over it can become dull to us.

"But," you ask, "if physical therapy is such a broad field with such a vast body of knowledge, how could that be boring? If every patient is different, how can that be boring?" Good questions.

In any PT setting, you will have some diversity of patients, but they still fall within a range. For instance, outpatient sports medicine clinics focus on orthopedic types of injuries, shoulder surgeries, knee replacements, and the like. Acute inpatient rehabilitation hospitals tend to have much lower level patients with severe limitations, but all within certain a spectrum of needs. Each setting markets to and attracts patients with the same types of conditions. Therapists tend to focus on a small part of the body of knowledge, gaining mastery of it within a short time. The challenge diminishes, especially if the area of practice is very narrow.

Even though all patients are different, each with their own unique personality, the truth is that therapists often have so many things to juggle that it is hard to have deep interaction with the people they are treating. As a therapist doing mostly evaluations and handing the daily treatment off to PTAs, this interaction is even more limited.

While there are several negative items on this list, please realize that a lot of therapists may not care about any of this at all. For example, it may not matter to some therapists if the corporate office tells them what to do. Plenty of people may love doing the same thing day after day. The pros for PT are very strong. The cons are bothersome to PTs, but even the most frustrated—including the PTs who leave the profession—will still keep their license current. It's peace of mind knowing you hold a piece of paper that will quickly get you a job making good money almost anywhere you want.

****

After this dose of negativity, now is a good time to pull out your list of affirmations and remind yourself what you want to accomplish!
****

Part 3

The First Decade

Chapter 10

Crawl, Walk, Run

GETTING YOUR FIRST JOB -- INTERVIEWS

Getting into physical therapy school is a very intense process. Programs use interviews to screen their applicants, and it's a good taste of what the real world will be like for job interviews. There is a significant difference, though: when there are lots of physical therapy jobs available, the applicant can evaluate the employer as well.

What does this mean? It means that physical therapy graduates need not feel as nervous with job interviews as they did with PT school interviews. Take it seriously? YES. Be so anxious that you sweat through your shirt? No. Why? Because you won't be competing against four hundred other students for a seat.

To lessen the anxiety, seek out multiple opportunities and interview with two or three of your top choices. Not only will this experience help you relax and gain confidence, but you will also likely receive multiple offers and get to take your top pick, and maybe even negotiate for a higher salary in the process.

There are many books available on the market that have helpful information about the interview process, although these are "general" interview books and are not specific to PT. As a new grad, your interviewer will probably ask about your clinical rotations and a few other things about PT school, but they are mostly trying to learn about your personality and decide how well you will fit into their workforce. If they are desperately seeking a PT, they may put on a full court press, trying to impress you enough that you will join their company. In either case, you will know plenty about PT for the interview, but it won't hurt to polish up your people skills or give a quick read through an interviewing book.

A book I highly recommend is *Salary Tutor* by Jim Hopkinson. Another great resource is a blog post by Ben Fung titled *5 Tips for Negotiating your Salary* (http://updocmedia.com/5-tips-for-negotiating-your-salary/), which I recommend reading if you want to know how to handle negotiations like a seasoned pro. Realize, though, that at this stage you're a new grad. Expect a job offer 20-25% below the average PT salaries for your area.

In the PT world negotiating salary is common, and the first offer you get will be low on purpose. Employers will expect you to counteroffer. If you push too much for higher pay then the employer could retract the offer (so, don't ask for $20,000 more). If you don't counteroffer then not only are you leaving money on the table, but you also could appear naive and even weak.

LEARNING TO CRAWL

YOU'RE HIRED! Congratulations! It's a great feeling to get out of PT school and start your first job!

Your first priority when you get out of school should be to master clinical competence. Getting off of the academic bus and out into the real world can be a big adjustment, especially if your first job is a little off the beaten path. As you travel away from metropolitan areas, the reality of PT practice can seem decades behind the cutting edge environment of a PT school.

Entering into a large workforce can have its own challenges, as well. Time management is a big hurdle for new PTs. Figuring out how to juggle problem patients, keep up with re-certifications, discharges, and getting your notes done and getting home before 6:00 p.m. is something every therapist has to master. Will you be delegating to PTAs? That is an art in and of itself. You will also want your billing to hit the right targets and keep your patients and doctors happy. All of this will soon be second nature, but for the first few months—unless you are completely unhappy with your job, your colleagues, your boss, or you are being asked to practice in an unethical or illegal way—stick with learning the craft of PT and don't worry about money.

I remember my first few weeks on the job as a new grad. The hospital rehab department had over thirty employees with physical, occupational, and speech therapists, physical therapist assistants, occupational therapist assistants, speech language pathologists, about ten aides or attendants, and three receptionists. All of the non-licensed folks had more hands-on experience than I did. Most of the staff was twice my age, and yet I was responsible for the patients I evaluated. I wasn't the manager, but it was my name on the paperwork, my license supporting the care we were providing. At the same time I was learning on the job every day from the PTAs and technicians I was supervising. It wasn't easy, and I didn't come through it unscathed, but I certainly didn't have time to think about money. You may not either in your first year or two.

ON YOUR FEET NOW

Once you have confidence in your new skills as a physical therapist, don't be afraid to start looking at options. Job opportunities abound! There are lots of ways to go about this, but it's all up to you. Be the captain of your own ship and explore.

Let's look at three ways you can increase your income during this period of time.

PRN Work. Not only will PRN work get you experience in new and different settings, broadening your experience and letting you learn what it would be like to work for another employer, PRNs can also earn very high hourly rates. How much money are we talking about? A common PRN rate is $50.00 per hour. If you can work two to three hours per week on a consistent basis, this can translate into $500 per month, or $6,000 per year. In some areas of the county rates can be much higher and can also include drive time. This can turn into $10,000 per year pretty quickly. Ask seasoned therapists about PRN opportunities in your area. Some companies might require one or two years of experience. Others might let you start earlier in your career. Find out how your current employer feels about you doing PRN work for another company. Not all will approve. Be professional and be open, but understand that doing PRN work for a competitor could be viewed unfavorably.

Change jobs. PT job opportunities abound in most areas of the country. As you gain experience, employers can offer salary increases anywhere from five to fifteen percent above your current gig. On average, therapists of all disciplines change jobs about every three to five years. Some will change jobs more frequently, others once every decade or so. Change too much and after ten years your resume will tell the story that: A) you're never satisfied, B) you're hard to work with, C) you don't make friends at work, or D) all of the above. Yes, opportunities abound. Yes, it is good and helpful to see if the grass is truly greener. But don't overdo it. Make a change and commit to it for a while. Changing jobs is scary, but keep in mind that your current employer will have no incentive to give you a strong salary increase if you do nothing.

The last two suggestions are essentially to work more or to change jobs. Perhaps neither of these appeals to you. Maybe you love your first job, the people there, and the mission of the organization, but you still want to increase your salary. There is a third option: **negotiate your pay.**

I'm going to share with you a passive-aggressive approach that employees have successfully used on me before, though it may not win you the respect of your boss--re-negotiate your pay with a written job offer from another employer. Here's how: line up an interview with another employer, something you genuinely think you'd like to do. This is important, because if your current employer calls your bluff you could have to take this job! Go to the interview, crush it, and get a job offer and maybe even a sign-on bonus offer. With your offer letter in writing, go to your current boss and break the news.

Your meeting with your boss might go something like this: "I'm thinking about trying something new, but I really like it here. Company X offered me this to go to work for them." Hold your ground at this point. Give time for the news to sink in. Hopefully you have a great relationship and your boss will say something like, "No! We don't want to lose you!" Or, if your time with your first job hasn't been great, it could be more like, "Well, best of luck, kid!" You should have a feel for it, but there's always room for surprises. This is why it's important that you really would enjoy working with the people who give you the job offer.

If your boss wants you to stay and you want to stay, you could say something like this: "Well, I'm torn. I want to stay, but this opportunity looks good. All things being equal, I'd probably stay. They did offer me more money, though." This is a passive-aggressive way of asking for a raise without coming right out and saying it. It's actually hiding the request for a raise behind the notion of wanting to try something different. I share it with you because it can work, though it leaves a bad taste in my mouth when an employee pulls this on me.

"Won't they be upset with me if I go interview somewhere else just to get a raise?" you ask. That depends on your true intentions and how much you show them. Don't be a jerk and you won't be treated like one. In the end, if you choose to stay with your employer, they will appreciate that they didn't lose you. Especially if you keep your raise to yourself.

This brings up an important point: talking about your salary with coworkers can be a fireable offense. Be careful.

One more thing before we move on. Try to interview to get a raise more than once with the same employer and your boss might just call your bluff. If it's an employers market, meaning therapists are easy to hire, then be certain you're ready to risk being shown the door before you try it. If therapists are hard to come by, the more likely it is that a second try will work.

It is possible to get a pay increase with a written offer letter in hand from somewhere else. Perhaps this is the strongest way to get your employer's attention, but it definitely sends a signal that you are ready and willing to leave, and it can tarnish your relationship with your boss and employer. The therapy world is small, and it could be a boss you don't like today could be the very person you want to work for in a decade. What if you really like where you work and you like your boss and you don't want to change jobs? Fortunately, there is another way.

Re-negotiate your pay without a written offer from another employer. Just as in patient care, each situation is different, and you need to consider several factors before deciding how to approach a renegotiation.

First, you need a firm understanding of what therapist salaries are in your area and industry, along with what you are generating for your current employer. There are lots of places where you can look at average salaries for different parts of the country, but volume and reimbursement rates determine why some PT settings pay more than others. If you are seeing a much higher volume than your colleagues in the same clinic you could use this to ask for higher pay. It is a completely different scenario if you are in line with or slightly behind everyone else.

Second, you need to understand the dynamics affecting your employer's ability to increase your salary. Is your clinic or department full of senior therapists who have been with the company for many years? If so, the business's therapist cost per patient will be high. In this scenario, the company has a stable and experienced staff and can hire another young therapist to fill your role. With the deck stacked against you like this, you may be less likely to get a raise. Is your clinic full of less experienced therapists, and is there a high turnover rate? Is your supervisor overwhelmed with treating patients and with management tasks? If so, you could be more likely to get a raise, especially if you are willing to help meet some needs for your employer. Realize that the higher a business's needs are, the more likely they will be to give you an increase if you meet those needs.

Third, you need to understand that all businesses, including healthcare, are in business to stay in business. This means your employer will want to pay you the lowest amount possible to keep you happy. You, on the other hand, are interested in earning every penny of what you feel you are worth. It's business, and while you may have a great relationship with your boss or clinic director, at the end of the day the business may not be able to give you what you want. Don't take it personally. It's business for them, too, and they won't take it personally if you ask for a raise, especially if you are professional and respectful of their situation.

Don't let fear stop you from asking! Unless you've had a bad run as an employee, your employer won't want to lose you. It can cost thousands of dollars in productivity to hire and train a new employee, which means it definitely can be worth it to pay you more. This gives you leverage, but business dynamics determine how much. Don't be afraid to have a conversation about your pay, but be courteous and be informed about everything we've covered so far.

Fourth, to increase your likelihood of success you should offer something that your employer needs that is of high value in exchange for the raise you are seeking. Yes, you could get more money and do nothing more, but if this is your motivation you should have a written offer in hand from someone else, as this strengthens your leverage. If you don't want to play that game, then offer value. You could, for instance, offer to work odd hours like late nights or weekends, or offer to take on a leadership role of some kind. Promise to deliver more than enough for your requested raise.

It's business. Sometimes you'll get what you want. Sometimes you won't. Be professional. Be courteous. No matter what the outcome, you'll benefit from going through a renegotiation experience.

"You don't always get what you want, but if you try sometime, you might just find, you get what you need." — The Rolling Stones

A PHYSICAL THERAPIST ON THE RUN!

Now you've been at it a while with no training wheels! Maybe you've had a couple of jobs, maybe more. You've been given raises and now make ten to twenty percent more than your first job. Guess what? Now you have even more opportunities, but the game changes.

Taking on more responsibility can open up more headroom for higher salaries. Become a department coordinator or a director and you could see a raise worth a few thousand dollars. Sometimes this comes in pay raises, and sometimes it comes with a bonus structure based on financial performance. Management of any kind always comes with extra work. If you are in a department with a lot of drama or if the workplace has a lot of political pressures, it easily could be that the extra money is not enough for the extra effort. If your increased pay is a bonus structure with unachievable goals, then you might just sign up for extra work and no extra pay.

Once, I was the regional manager over three nursing homes. Two of them were fairly close together, but it was an hour and a half drive between the two that were farthest apart. My job was to coordinate about 30 staff members—some full-time and lots of PRN staff—to get all of the patients evaluated within 24 hours of their admission. A very popular time for nursing home admissions is Friday afternoon, and it was always hard to find therapists willing to work a couple of hours at the end of their work week. It was my responsibility to make sure our company provided care for every patient according to the guidelines of our contracts. If I couldn't get help to do evaluations, who do you think had to do them? That's right—me. That meant driving an hour and a half to see a patient admitted on a Friday afternoon at 5:30pm, having thirty minutes or more of evaluation and documentation time, and then having over an hour's drive home. All for no extra money.

A friend had a management job with income incentives in the form of quarterly bonuses. Her targets were set once a year during budgetary planning. Budgets are great, but it's hard to foresee everything that can happen in a year. And even if you know something substantial is coming it can be very hard to predict the full effect of forces beyond the manager's control. One year she did great. The next year was a different story. None of it was within her control, but she didn't hit her targets. The result: missed bonuses and less pay than the previous year to the tune of twelve thousand dollars.

If you choose to pursue the management route, just be sure that management is what you want and that you are comfortable with your pay structure.

Are there opportunities besides management? Absolutely. That's what the rest of this book is about. There's one more thing for us to cover that all therapists need to understand: there is an income ceiling.

Chapter 11

Hitting the Ceiling

"Clap along if you feel like a room without a roof." —
Pharrel Williams

If you've been working as a therapist for a decade or so, then the fact that there is a ceiling for income is no surprise. Yes, it's possible to change jobs and get raises easily for ten years. As we have said before, after this amount of time there are usually fewer job opportunities that inspire you, and if you check into these jobs you'll find that they don't offer more money.

Why does this happen?

We'll have to explore a little more about business in healthcare to see it. Let's go up and see the big picture from 30,000 feet.

Remember our basic business formula: Profit = Income - Overhead

Where does income come from in physical therapy? In over 95% of cases, it comes from insurance companies. Over the past three decades, reimbursement within all of medicine has slowly declined. Hospitals are paid less for helping someone get over pneumonia, surgeons are paid less for performing a knee replacement, and therapists are paid less for helping a person who had a stroke relearn to walk.

How is it that an entire industry is paid less today than it was thirty years ago? That requires us to go up to 60,000 feet.

Most insurance companies base their rates on the Medicare Fee Schedule. Whatever the tax-base funded, government-managed insurance company does, goes. If Medicare decides it needs to pay doctors and hospitals and everyone else in healthcare 1% less, they do, and healthcare providers have no recourse. "Thank you very much," is all there is to say. Then, when everyone in healthcare has no option but to take less reimbursement from Medicare, all of the other insurance companies follow suit.

How is this okay? Let's go up one more time, to 90,000 feet.

Our country has more and more people reaching the age to receive Medicare benefits, enough that more money is going out than what is coming in. For years, evangelists have been preaching that reform was needed, that if we didn't change we would reach a point where the system failed. Small corrections were put in place in the form of a schedule of annual incremental decreases to provider reimbursement. The Medicare Sustainable Growth Rate (SGR) was a method used by the Centers for Medicare and Medicaid Services (CMS) in the United States to control spending by Medicare on physician services.

This sounds positive for the government and for the social issues that we face as a nation, but it is a big problem for providers. In the past fifteen years the trend has been for Congress to pass a "patch" to stop the decreases from occurring. Each year the patch kept a 1-2% decrease from occurring, but the underlying legislation that held the schedule of incremental decreases was left in place. Each year the gap between where this legislation called for Medicare rates to be and where they actually were held grew larger and larger, until in 2015 it was 21%.

In 2015, Congressional action finally repealed the SGR. New legislation provided small increases in healthcare reimbursement, but they did not "fix" the system. As a nation we are still faced with the problem of having many aging Americans entering the Medicare system and not enough money to cover their medical expenses.

Remember that what we're talking about is why reimbursement is declining. Medicare is a large part of it, but it's not the entire story.

The Affordable Care Act of 2014 affected private insurance companies and forced them to provide coverage to Americans with pre-existing conditions. It also established a National Exchange where several different insurance plans are available for purchase and where tax incentives make insurance affordable to individuals and families with low incomes. Both of these are very positive.

There is a negative side, though. Patients with pre-existing conditions usually have many claims. Translation: high costs. The government said that private health insurance carriers have to take on this population, but insurance companies are businesses too, and income has to exceed overhead to stay in business.

How will this income be generated? Multiple fronts. The premiums that businesses pay to give their employees insurance coverage have gone up tremendously after the Affordable Care Act was passed. What's more, many plans with lower premiums have very high deductibles. A three thousand dollar deductible means that if a patient has shoulder surgery, a procedure that will most certainly cost over three thousand dollars, the patient will have to pay for their entire surgery out of their own pocket, and the insurance company would only pay the amount that exceeds the deductible. The majority of people have low medical expenses each year, and high deductibles shift the costs for the majority away from insurance companies.

Are there good intentions with high deductible plans? Yes. Consumers who have to pay a large amount to have a test or procedure performed will be more inclined to evaluate what they are getting for their money, and might even choose not to have the test or procedure if it is not absolutely necessary. The downside of this is that patients may put off getting care they need because they would rather not spend several hundred dollars on it.

Now, returning to our quest to understand why there is a ceiling in PT salaries. Medicare isn't going to pay providers more. Private insurance companies are not raising their reimbursement rates. What's more, they have shifted a significant portion of financial responsibility to the patient, making them consumers within healthcare, and at the same time have made it more difficult for providers to get paid since they have to collect from patients directly. The bottom line is, the picture of healthcare reimbursement from 30,000, 60,000, and 90,000 feet isn't pretty. Given all of this, it is safe to say that providers at all levels are unlikely to see raises in reimbursement anytime soon.

Physical therapists are in business all across the country, though. They are still making money, right? Yes, of course. But no medical provider that bills insurance companies is able to control how much they will be paid for a billable unit of service.

The components of income that are more in our control are volume and the payer mix of insurance companies within that volume.

Let's first consider volume. Remember our discussion about physician referrals? Some states don't require a referral from a physician in order to initiate physical therapy, but most insurances still do. Physical therapists have to establish good working relationships with physicians in order to get enough referrals to keep their volumes high. Lose a relationship, lose referrals. In spite of many years of learning resulting in doctorate level education, physical therapists still have to work to keep physicians happy to keep their businesses healthy.

What if there is all the volume in the world? It's a good problem to have. Still, there is a limit on the number of patients a physical therapist can see. Once, it was common for therapists to have fifteen to twenty patients on their schedules each day. Insurance regulations have restricted how much time a therapist has to spend with an individual patient in order to bill for a unit of service, and more documentation is required to get paid. Now it is more common for therapists to see twelve patients during an eight-hour day, and with that it can be very hard to finish all of the notes by quitting time.

Reimbursement rates are not in our control, and there is a ceiling on volume, but within the socioeconomic limitations of a community, providers can work to have a strong payer mix. A therapy business in a wealthy part of town will likely have a high concentration of patients with insurance that pays well. It's also likely that wealthier patients will have less difficulty paying their deductibles. The converse to this is unfortunately true. Areas with more poverty are likely to have patients with no insurance or insurance that reimburses poorly. They also can be less able to pay high deductibles.

Location, location, location, right? Yes, but patients are not stationary. Physical therapy business has a strong referral component. Excellent work can earn a reputation where physicians refer to certain physical therapy businesses no matter where they are. Still, there is a limit to this. While increasing the concentration of a top-paying insurance and limiting the patients seen with lower paying insurance can have a noticeable effect, moving this beyond a few percentage points is difficult to achieve and sustain.

Now we have covered the major components to income: therapists can't control reimbursement rates, there is a ceiling on volume per therapist, and there is only so much that can be changed with payer mix. Now let's look further at overhead.

Profit = Income - Overhead

Of course, the world around us has gotten more expensive. Thirty years ago, having a computer within a business was uncommon; now it is a requirement, along with a high-speed Internet connection and software with a monthly license fee. The cost of employee benefits is going up (remember our discussion of the Affordable Care Act?), as is the cost of advertising, utility services, laundry service, uniforms, equipment, and a million other small business items. It's simply more expensive to stay in business.

Any business that has employees knows this is true: every year they will want a raise. The world we live in is getting more expensive, and it takes more money to maintain a certain lifestyle.

How can healthcare businesses survive if they have limited ability to control income and overhead continues to rise? It's not easy. Difficult choices have to be made. Staff raises get spread out to once every two to three years. Rather than 3-5% raises, which were common ten years ago, 1-2% raises are the norm today. Businesses are shopping for cheaper services in an attempt to save money. Cheaper insurance, different supply providers, lowering phone bills—all of these things can lower overhead to some degree.

There is another big way to lower overhead that isn't so pleasant: hire less expensive staff.

The cheapest therapy staff available are new graduates. Primed with new knowledge and eager to begin treating patients, new graduates can be a great way to pump enthusiasm into a business. The downside: unless there is upward mobility within an organization, and good raises to boot, new graduates are tempted by the many opportunities available to them within a couple of years.

The ideal therapist has two to three years of experience, solid skills as a PT, is able to integrate into the workforce, is able to do the same work as an experienced therapist and get reimbursed the same from insurance companies, and most importantly, is not as expensive as a person with ten years of experience.

Here is a reality about insurance reimbursement in physical therapy that is sad but true: it doesn't matter who performs a unit of service—a new graduate, a physical therapist assistant, or a PT with multiple certifications and more than twenty years of experience—insurance companies will reimburse the very same amount.

When income is fixed, businesses will realize more profit by lowering overhead. No, they can't get away with firing senior staff because they are senior, but they don't have to keep giving raises. The sad truth is, companies don't want to lose you, but they don't have to keep paying you more.

Can you say, "Hello, income ceiling?"

****

Reminder — Where are you with your 30-Day Challenge? "Why" *are you interested in more income as a PT? What are you doing to make yourself worthy of higher income?*
****

RECERTIFICATION

SUBJECTIVE: Reader presents today having achieved much with this book to this point. A toolbox has been filled, the state of PT salaries in today's world is understood, as well as the typical progress that can be seen in the first decade of practice.

OBJECTIVE: Findings show that the reader still needs an understanding of basic income principles, and will also benefit from in-depth examples of different opportunities for increasing income.

ASSESSMENT: Continued physical therapy is warranted to progress toward the following, updated goals:

1. Read through the following section with information about income strategies, and gain mastery of the principles of "slowlane" and "fastlane" income generation in Chapter 12 before proceeding to Chapters 13 and 14.

2. Discover ten interviews with entrepreneurs and business leaders in Part 4.

3. Continue with 30-Day Challenge, Daily Routines, and Sharing with colleagues and with the PTCSG Community.

PLAN: Continue with the rest of this book, and reach out to all of the interviewees to thank them for their contributions.

Part 4

Raise the Ceiling

Chapter 12

Slowlane and Fastlane

Before we get into the nitty gritty of raising the income ceiling, it is important to discuss a few principles of income production.

One time, the practice I worked for bought lunch for a physician's practice, and hundreds of dollars of food from a top caterer stretched down the hall on folding tables. Plates in hand, a doctor talked with me about a prime plot of land he owned that was next to our clinic.

"Yeah, I want to clear that lot and put in a doughnut shop or something," he said. This was interesting, but his next sentence grabbed onto something deep inside of me. I think it still might be ringing in my head.

"I want to build something that will make money while I'm sleeping."

Here I was talking to a doctor who probably made three times what I made as a clinic director, but he wanted to supplement his lifestyle with a different *type* of income stream.

All that I have learned of revenues and income in the years since this moment has only reinforced the revelation that hit me that day: healthcare is a hands-on business that requires a provider to be there working in order to make money. There are other types of businesses that bring in money in different ways. This may seem like a no-brainer, but it was a brand new way of thinking about making money for me.

The doctor was talking about *passive income*. Passive income describes a type of business that produces revenue without the owner's daily presence and involvement. Some people seek passive income for the lifestyle it affords, some seek it to stabilize their income, and some seek multiple passive income streams that will provide them with money for retirement. There are as many legitimate reasons for this as there are types of businesses. Some common examples of passive income include: rental property, billboard advertising (the billboards themselves, not the advertising), vending machines, investing, writing books, and a whole host of online businesses. All of these require upfront work (sometimes a lot), and then, when you get the mix just right, the money flows.

We aren't going to praise passive income as the "be-all, end-all" of income, but it opens the door to a much larger topic of how therapists make money.

We have already made the point that physical therapy—and healthcare in general—is a field that trades time for money. Therapists have to treat patients in order to generate revenue. We get a pretty good exchange—not in the same ballpark as what an orthopedic surgeon gets, but a good deal more than unskilled labor. That's not the point. That's not the reason you're reading this book.

There's a rub, and we all know it. Some therapists recognize it and do something about it. Others feel it, but don't know how to call it by name, or know how to escape it.

The ceiling on physical therapist pay is related to how many hours in a week we can work. Yes, a huge factor in our income levels is what hourly rate of reimbursement our business gets paid for our work. Yes, the overhead in our business can eat away profits. Yes, a steady stream of referrals is needed to keep it all stable. Even with all of these set to optimal levels, however, therapists can only see a certain number of patients per day. Our main limit, and the number one reason why therapists' salaries don't continue to rise after ten years of practice, is that we only have so much time to trade for money.

MJ DeMarco penned a landmark book called *The Millionaire Fastlane*. In my opinion, this book is **must-read** material for anyone who wants to understand income better. In the book, DeMarco describes the trade of time for money as a "Slowlane" approach to wealth. This is a better strategy than being on the "Sidewalk," where people use debt to borrow against the future to have a life of instant gratification; the sidewalk's destination is being poor. In the Slowlane, people trade time for money, budget aggressively, and depend on compounding interest for their future wealth. Forty years of working and saving might provide a nice retirement, but there are risks: the freedom of retirement comes late in life, and we aren't guaranteed fifteen healthy years from sixty-five to eighty; the stock market could crash right before we retire, which would radically alter our lifestyle in the sunset of life; and while on the journey, we have to suffer through the trials of having a job.

The distinction between "Fastlane" and "Slowlane" will come up repeatedly in the rest of this book, so let's dive a little deeper.

As anyone who has had a job can attest, jobs have their downside. Workers have limited leverage (being fifty percent more productive won't get you a fifty percent raise), and limited control (companies fail, companies have layoffs, bad bosses abound). Workers are subject to the whims of their employer, they have to deal with office politics, and they have almost no control over their incomes.

Want to escape all of this by climbing the management ladder? Consider this quote by Robert Frost: "By working faithfully eight hours a day you may eventually get to be boss and work twelve hours a day."

Slowlane workers, even the ones who have their own businesses, are limited by the time for money constraint. If you want to earn twenty percent more you have to work twenty percent more. You could double your work hours and be miserable, but there is no way to work ten times more.

There are many reasons why a person might want to choose the Fastlane, but the main three DeMarco describes are: family, fitness, and freedom. Being wealthy is not all about money. Physical therapists cringe at the idea of being "all about the money." To DeMarco, having wealth means being healthy, being surrounded by great friends and family, and having the freedom to live life the way you want to live it.

Physical therapy provides most of these things. Generally, it's a first-shift job, giving nights and weekends off for personal time and family. You can easily get a job anywhere you want and have good income, but the "time for money" issue limits freedom.

According to DeMarco, the Fastlane uses controllable but unlimited leverage for growth. Success needs to be scalable to allow a one hundred or even one thousand percent return. With five to ten years of focused and accountable work, a high level of wealth can be achieved that gives freedom to life. The Fastlane doesn't avoid work, but it focuses on building systems that do the work, optimizing and automating relentlessly. It shifts focus from being a consumer to being a producer, from being a person who buys a franchise to being the person who sells franchises, from being a person who buys late-night infomercial products to a person producing and selling them.

Physical therapy is a service profession. The work of a single physical therapist has a limited scale and fits into the Slowlane category. There are ways to overcome this, plenty of which are on full display in the therapy world. Different business structures cope with scale in different ways, making them Fastlane income sources for business owners.

In addition to providing higher income that fuels lifestyles, Fastlane strategies have another significant benefit: businesses can be sold for strong profits.

There is a debate in the field at large about who is an entrepreneur. Some say that because they own their own business that they are entrepreneurs. Others argue that scale is needed in order to claim the entrepreneurial title. Who is right? The answer may hinge on if the business is considered a Fastlane business. Another considerable point of distinction are business exit strategies. What makes a business one that can be sold? In an article in *PPS Impact Magazine*, Franklin J. Rooks Jr, PT, MBA, Esq. gives a great answer:

"What do you have to sell? Some practice owners have been met with a rude awakening when they realize that they do not have anything to sell. That is, what they have built [their business] is not of value to any would-be buyer. As many practitioners have come to see, there is a tremendous distinction in the creation of a job versus the creation of a business. Many private practitioners have outstanding clinical expertise and provide exceptional care, but that alone does not create a business. Many practitioners have been able to set up shop, design their own hours, control their vacation times, answer to themselves, and practice physical therapy the way they want. They are their own bosses. Unless there is a significant earnings number created in the process, the private practitioner has succeeded in creating a job for him/ herself. Instead of working for a hospital or other entity, the practitioner has chosen to work for him/herself. This is laudable, but not worthy of any financial consideration as part of any value-added transaction. Acquirers are not purchasing jobs, they are purchasing businesses."

What Franklin Rooks is describing is the difference between the Slowlane and the Fastlane. Yes, physical therapists can own their own businesses and control their own hours and make good money. Unless the business makes a strong profit beyond what the owner makes by his or her own work, though, it is a Slowlane job. Fastlane businesses make money whether the owner is there or not, and they create profit that will interest acquirers. This brings us to a very important principle that can have tremendous implications for therapists.

Before anything can be sold it has to have a value. For used cars there is the *Kelley Blue Book*. In the real estate business, recent comparable sales are figured into the value of a house. Businesses are different and have to be calculated based on a number of factors.

Perhaps the most important valuation measure of a business is called EBITDA. This term is an acronym for yearly earnings before interest, taxes, depreciation, and amortization. It is a purer method of looking at a business's earning potential than just net income. There are several ways of calculating EBITDA, and in some situations it is not an accurate predictor of business value, but it is commonly used to determine a very important factor for business sale.

EBITDA is a measure of a business's yearly earning potential, but not its selling price. As with anything, the selling price of a business is negotiable, but formulas used to reach a value multiply EBITDA by a "multiple." For instance, if EBITDA is a value of $750,000 and the multiplier is 4.5, the business value is $3,375,000. Multiples vary from industry to industry, but within physical therapy they usually range from 2 to 12, depending on a number of metrics that determine the strength of the business (location, payer mix, visits per referral, leadership, etc.).

A very large physical therapy firm was recently acquired at a rumored multiple of 13. If this is true, and if debt didn't erase the gains, then it was an enormous payday for the business owners and investors.

Optimizing metrics and scale in the years preceding acquisition is common for business owners. While in some cases this can seem distasteful to employees, it is a common Fastlane tactic used to balloon the business's valuation at just the right time.

We're scratching the surface here, but Joseph LaPorta has a great article with more detail on metrics and exit plans that can be found on the WebPT blog.
https://www.webpt.com/blog/post/mastering-metrics-exit

Building any business takes time and effort and requires risk-taking, but not all business types will produce the same end result. Just as it is important to know your 'why'—why you go into a certain business, why you take a particular path—it is ***equally important to understand the impact 'what' type of business you choose to build will have on exit strategies***.

As we move forward and look at ways physical therapists can raise their income ceiling, we will discuss several components to business structure:

- Required overhead
- Financial risks
- Revenue opportunity
- Slowlane vs Fastlane
- "Time for Money" vs. Passive Income
- Scale
- Time frame to success
- Long-term potential for higher income
- Potential for business sale at exit

For each of these we'll apply a five point scoring method for how it relates to raising therapist income.

Highly Unfavorable ->
Unfavorable ->
Neutral ->
Favorable ->
Highly Favorable ->

We'll also discuss why each score is given.

With most types of structures, we will talk with entrepreneur physical therapists who have built this type of business. Their wisdom and experiences will illustrate what can be accomplished with hard work and focused discipline.

The therapy world is broad and wide. Just as there are some people who are over seven feet tall, I'm sure there will be exceptions to the things we will discuss in the next section. Please seek professional business advice when needed, and make choices for your own career path with the same care that you give to your patients.

Chapter 13

Opportunities in Standard PT Practice

"You don't have to be great to start, but you have to start to be great." —Zig Ziglar

Realizing that there is no more headroom for increased income can be depressing. Unfortunately, this awareness usually comes after several years in the profession, when the rewards of providing care can be diminished, when life can be in full swing, and when extra money would be useful. With this awareness, we immediately notice all of the other therapists we know who took entrepreneurial career paths and who are now making more money, some with expanding income potential. The more you are paying attention to income, the more the ceiling will seem lower and lower, and the practice of physical therapy can become less and less rewarding.

For those of us who have reached this point, wouldn't it have been great if someone had told us this was coming? Wouldn't it have been great if at five or six years into our career someone had pulled us aside and told us about opportunities within the profession where therapists could direct their careers and avoid income ceilings? Wouldn't it have been nice to have known how to steer your career toward the potential for higher earnings?

Well, there's no time like the present.

PRN Work

One of the easiest ways for a therapist to have increased income is PRN work. PRN means "as needed." For therapists, "as needed" can be almost all the time. Nursing homes, school systems, rural hospitals, and home health agencies often need help with evaluations and treatments, but they don't have enough need to justify hiring additional full-time staff.

How much money are we talking about? Let's do some math. A common PRN rate is $50.00 per hour. If a therapist is able to work two to three hours per week on a consistent basis, this can translate into $500.00 per month, and $6,000 per year. Some therapists have multiple PRN jobs. Rates can be $75 per hour, and even include travel to and from facilities. This can turn into $10,000 per year pretty quickly.

PRN work can be a great way to test out a different area of practice, though some general experience is needed. For instance, a therapist working in acute care probably would have no difficulty providing PRN coverage at a long-term care facility, but a therapist working in home health might not be as comfortable providing PRN help for a school system. It all depends on each therapist's background and experience, and how much assistance and training will come from the employer.

This brings us to a component of current practice that somewhat limits PRN work: documentation. Most businesses have shifted to electronic charting. While many of the principles of documenting remain constant in any area of practice, each electronic medical record system is different. It can take a while to learn and gain proficiency with some systems. If the area of practice has additional requirements, as home health does, then knowing how to document can be a high hurdle that could limit some PRN opportunities.

Most companies want PRN therapists with a year or two of experience. This experience requirement might be less if you are working in the same area of practice as your first job. If you have some months of solid work under your belt, start asking around about PRN opportunities.

A note of caution here: your employer may not want you to do PRN work for other companies. In some settings and in some positions, doing work for other businesses is frowned upon. This is especially true if the PRN job is with a competitor. The first place you go to learn about PRN opportunities in your area probably does not need to be your boss. Most therapists with ten years of experience have had one or more PRN jobs—start there with your questions.

One more word of caution: depending on your relationship with your employer and your desire to stay long-term in your current job, you should strongly consider telling your supervisor that you are going to do PRN work. This is a common thing for therapists to do, and even if it isn't liked, you will be respected for your openness. You might even be asked to bring back good ideas to share. Every situation is different. Some employers may require employees to acknowledge conflicts of interest. Know your risks, and be professional.

PRN jobs are wonderful ways to make extra money. Just as therapy jobs are almost everywhere, so are PRN jobs. With them, you can test out different areas of practice to see how well you like them without changing jobs; you can work with a company for a few weeks or a few months and gain insight into their management principles and decide if you like working with their staff; you can learn a new medical record system (which, believe it or not, is a good thing); and you can see how well working extra hours fits into your life.

The downside of income that comes from PRN work is that it is a time for money exchange. You can layer on extra income, but if you ever have to stop doing PRN work or if the employer stops using you, the money stops flowing. An additional negative is that the additional money is not really a salary increase, and the time required to make the extra money is time lost to developing passive income.

PRN Work "Raise the Ceiling" Scores:

Required Overhead — Highly Favorable. Usually there are no costs or very low costs to provide PRN work for another company. No costs means the money you make is yours to keep.

Financial Risks — Highly Favorable. All that is at risk in PRN work is your own time. You could have additional liability risks, but usually your PRN employer has liability coverage for all of their therapists. If this is something you fear, HPSO (Healthcare Providers Service Organization) provides low-cost liability insurance plans that will give you additional personal coverage.

Revenue Opportunity — Favorable. You only have to perform the work of a therapist when you do PRN work. No business skills are needed, and you make a very high rate while you're at it. The reason this isn't "highly favorable" is that money from PRN work is limited by time.

Slowlane vs. Fastlane — Slowlane

"Time for Money" vs. Passive Income — Unfavorable. If you aren't working, you aren't making money. Get sick or go on vacation and the money stops. The advantage of PRN work is that the hourly rate is usually good, but this doesn't change the fact that it is a time for money exchange.

Scale — Highly Unfavorable. There's just one of you, and there are only so many hours in a week.

Time Frame To Success — Highly Favorable. If you start doing PRN work you'll probably get an extra paycheck within a few weeks. Extra money in your pocket — POW!

Long-Term Potential for Increased Income — Neutral. PRN work is not guaranteed, nor is a therapist's energy or desire to work extra hours. It can be done, though, and there are abundant opportunities. If one PRN job dries up, then a therapist who wants the income will have to look for another. Remember, we are talking about a few thousand dollars a year. This is good fun money, but it isn't going to triple your income.

Potential for Sale at Exit — Highly Unfavorable. There is nothing to sell.

	PRN Work
Required Overhead	Highly Favorable
Financial Risks	Highly Favorable
Revenue Opportunity	Favorable
Slowlane vs. Fastlane	Slowlane
"Time for Money" vs. Passive Income	Unfavorable
Scale	Highly Unfavorable
Time Frame to Success	Highly Favorable
Longterm Potential for Increased Income	Neutral
Potential for Sale at Exit	Highly Unfavorable

Specialization and Certification

I'm going to do it—I'm going to tread on thin ice here.

Physical therapy has different specialties where a therapist can achieve certification. These usually come in the form of completing several continuing education units in succession and passing an exam. The knowledge and experience gained from these programs can be extensive. Becoming a certified therapist in any genre can be very rewarding both in completing the process itself and in the prestige garnered by having the certification.

Know this, though: insurance companies do not care if a therapist is certified.

Yes, therapists with specialized certification are more marketable because of the evidence of their competence. Yes, therapists with certifications are strong members of any clinic because of their ability to take on challenging patients with problems that stump less experienced staff. Yes, certification proves within the medical community that a therapist has expert level knowledge of a given subset of physical therapy, and this could bring in more referrals. Yes, companies appreciate certification and will try harder to retain a therapist with specialized training. All of these things are true, which means that certification can bring a therapist more income.

It can, but not always. Slowlaners believe that education is the way to raise their value. It just doesn't always happen.

As we have already said, insurance companies do not pay more for a unit of therapy if a certified person performs it. It's all the same to payers. No matter how much skill or training or expertise went into a unit of manual therapy or therapeutic exercise, they are going to pay the same amount to the business. This is the major reason certification does not always bring increased income.

Another reason certification may not be beneficial is because many clinics treat generalized populations. A certified manual therapist who only has one or two patients a week that require specialized care is not utilizing this knowledge in a way that warrants extra pay.

If you take away honor, rank, prestige, and the joy of having specialized training and deep understanding, and you look instead at the financial impact that certification programs bring verses the time, energy, and expense to achieve that certification, you would both cringe *and be excited.*

Wait a minute...what?

It's true. In the therapy world at large, certification will usually only bring a slight increase in pay for therapists. Most of the time, employers will not pay extra for therapists to get certification. However, there are situations in "niche markets" where specialization can make all the difference in the world. Golf, tennis, and running are examples of areas where clients may seek performance enhancement training by those certified in sports physical therapy.

Specialization and Certification "Raise the Ceiling" Scores:

Required Overhead — Slightly Unfavorable to Neutral. Therapists must have so many continuing education units each year to maintain licensure. These can be directed toward a certification path. However, many certifications require multiple courses, and spreading the learning out over several years may not be ideal. The cost of completing the certification in a shorter timeframe may exceed employer benefits for reimbursement and time off work for continuing education. This extra expense will be the therapist's responsibility. Months of work and thousands of dollars of expense will offset any raise that comes with certification.

Financial Risk — Neutral. It can take extra money to gain a certification, but not all the rewards for going through the process are monetary.

Revenue Opportunity — This one ranges from Unfavorable to Favorable. Some certifications give therapists skills needed to perform tasks that are beyond the scope of general therapy. Some of these tasks are highly profitable. A therapist with a high concentration of highly profitable tasks can generate more revenue and have a higher chance of increased income (for example, a therapist trained to conduct NCV exams). A therapist with a certification working in a generalized therapy clinic will not bring any more revenue to the business and likely will not make more money.

Slowlane vs. Fastlane — Slowlane

"Time for Money" vs. Passive Income — Highly Unfavorable. Certification does not change the time for money exchange. If no increased income is realized after obtaining the certification, then the therapist has spent time and energy to obtain education that does not provide a monetary reward. Money isn't everything, and it isn't the only reward, but our focus is raising income ceilings.

Scale — Very Unfavorable. There's just one of you, and there are only so many hours in a week for you to use a certification.

Time Frame To Success — Unfavorable. Certifications and Specializations are not easy to achieve, and they may or may not bring immediate financial rewards. For therapists who wish to raise their income quickly, the time and energy and money spent on certification could be spent on activities with higher potential to increase earnings. It is worth noting, however, that certifications could the be the pathway to earning greater respect within the professional community, paving the way for teaching and educating opportunities that we will discuss in the next chapter.

Potential for Sale at Exit — Highly Unfavorable. There is nothing to sell.

	Specialization and Certification
Required Overhead	Neutral
Financial Risks	Neutral
Revenue Opportunity	Neutral
Slowlane vs. Fastlane	Slowlane
"Time for Money" vs. Passive Income	Highly Unfavorable
Scale	Highly Unfavorable
Time Frame to Success	Highly Unfavorable
Longterm Potential for Increased Income	Highly Unfavorable
Potential for Sale at Exit	Highly Unfavorable

Private Practice Outpatient Clinics

Why work for someone else when you can open your own clinic and have other therapists work for you? Oh, if it were only that easy.

There are many challenges facing therapists who open private practice clinics. Depending on the location, competition can be strong, facility overhead can be high, and therapists can be difficult to recruit and retain. On top of this is the difficulty of collecting payment from insurance companies; the costs of marketing, technology, and employee benefits; and the threat of a competitor with deep pockets moving in and taking away your referral base.

All the risks of starting any business are inherent in opening a physical therapy practice. A recent sad story tells how a young therapist paid $250,000 to buy a practice from a retiring therapist. She couldn't keep it going. The business closed within a few months, but she still had the bank note to pay off.

Two major factors that make it difficult to start a private practice are location and competition. We'll take each in turn.

Location. Remember how we said earlier that physicians drive physical therapy business? That comes into play here. Several things about location drive volume: the impression that patients and referral sources get from the clinic itself, the proximity to referral sources and to patients, and the ease of access to get in and out of the building. Get all of this right at a price tag your clinic can support and you could have gold mine. The more competition there is, the more these things matter. Here's a caveat: you can skimp on any of the location/facility items if your referral source is consistent and loyal, or if you have no competition. The converse is also true: if your referral source is not loyal you can own the Taj Mahal and it won't matter.

Competition. The better the location, the more it will attract competition. Competition dilutes volume, raises marketing costs, makes the impression of the facility that much more important, and gives therapists other employment options. Large corporations are able to place new clinics in ideal locations knowing it can take years for them to be profitable. This financial backing enables them to outlast individual therapists. When the competition is a new physician-owned clinic, referrals can disappear almost overnight.

Let's not forget the effects of decreasing reimbursement and increased effort needed to collect. Every corner of healthcare is touched by this. Fighting for referrals, fighting for reimbursement, fighting to hire therapists, fighting to retain therapists—it's easy to see why more and more private practices are selling to large corporations or going out of business.

Those that are able to weather the storms of the present day are usually well-established practices in prime locations with strong reputations in their patient and referral base. Facility debt has been paid down over many years, thus lowering both overhead and risk for practice owners. Those with expanded operations and multiple locations have the power of centralized operations and can be more profitable to the owners.

New therapist-owned private practices that are successful have to navigate these waters with great care. Where and how are they successful? That's what we'll talk about next. (If you're thinking that this is too short of a section for private practice—not to worry—the next two sections focus on specializations within private practice.)

Private Practice Outpatient Clinic "Raise the Ceiling" Scores:

Required Overhead — Unfavorable to Highly Unfavorable. This can depend on the type of business, but most general outpatient PT practices have large footprints and expensive exercise equipment. This will be more expensive if the facility is in a prime location.

Financial Risks — Unfavorable to Highly Unfavorable. The more you spend on overhead, the more is at risk. The better the location, the more likely it is that a competitor will come in and take away market share.

Revenue Opportunity — Neutral. Physical therapy is a profitable business, however margins are getting tighter and tighter, and risks are substantial. The balance of required overhead and revenue opportunity should be evaluated very closely before making any business decision, particularly when opening an outpatient private practice.

Slowlane vs. Fastlane — Slowlane, with potential to move toward Fastlane. If a business owner is able to expand the clinic to have multiple therapists and multiple locations, then this is moving toward Fastlane.

"Time for Money" vs. Passive Income — Unfavorable. Outpatient private practices do not change the time for money issue common to physical therapy.

Scale — Unfavorable to Highly Favorable. Therapy businesses are complicated. If you are working 'in" the business as well as the person who works "on" the business, then growing can be difficult. If the market is strong enough for a clinic to expand its operations, then this can be favorable. Fastlane is expanding to multiple clinics and large scale.

Time Frame To Success — Unfavorable. Depending on the success of marketing, it can take months to fill up a therapist's schedule. Factor in the necessary overhead involved to run the business and it may take many more months to reach profitability.

Long-Term Potential for Increased Income — Favorable. If outside and uncontrollable forces do not negatively impact the business, outpatient private practices can be profitable. Many elements play into this: how well the business is run, how well overhead is managed, how many patients are seen each week, and if there are multiple locations. Keep in mind that many outpatient practices are being sold to large corporations, which might be exactly what you want at some point in your career.

One or Two Locations Potential for Sale at Exit — Neutral to Favorable. Is the business in a good location, with a strong payer mix, solid leadership beneath the owner(s), and with low competition and a history of profitability? These things raise the potential for an acquisition. If the business is marginal, and especially if the owner is the main therapist, this potential is much lower.

Large, Multi-Location Potential for Sale at Exit — Favorable to Highly Favorable. Many more metrics will determine the multiple at sale, but larger businesses have potential for revenue generation that will attract investors.

	Private Practice Outpatient - Single/small company	Private Practice Outpatient - Large Scale
Required Overhead	Highly Unfavorable	Highly Unfavorable
Financial Risks	Highly Unfavorable	Highly Unfavorable
Revenue Opportunity	Neutral	Neutral
Slowlane vs. Fastlane	Slowlane	Fastlane
"Time for Money" vs. Passive Income	Unfavorable	Unfavorable
Scale	Neutral	Highly Favorable
Time Frame to Success	Unfavorable	Unfavorable
Longterm Potential for Increased Income	Favorable	Highly Favorable
Potential for Sale at Exit	Neutral	Highly Favorable

Niche Markets

One of the buzzwords in the therapy world for the last twenty years has been "niche markets." By definition, niche means "a specialized but profitable corner of the market." With declining revenues all around, it's no wonder that anything that is profitable is all the rage.

So, what makes a niche market within physical therapy?

The first element we want to consider is "profitable." There are certain constraints to physical therapy, no matter what arena. All reimbursement is regulated by insurance company fee schedules and by their time-bound rules and guidelines. For a practice to be profitable as it compares to the therapy world at large, it will have one of two qualities: either it will have the ability to keep longer hours of operation, thereby providing more units of treatment to more patients than average, or it will have a very concentrated payer mix or alternate payment source that results in substantially higher collections per charged unit than average.

Clinics in urban areas have populations that work all hours of the day and night. To meet the needs of patients in these areas, there are physical therapy clinics that have two or more shifts of therapists so they can offer expanded hours of operation. You might be thinking that this doesn't sound like specialization, and it's not in the sense of certification within physical therapy. Think about this, though: most clinics do not stay open beyond ten to eleven hours a day. A well run, twenty-four hour a day physical therapy practice can be very profitable because it will have high total volume and low equipment and building overhead relative to each hour of performed care.

Expanding hours of operation can have the same effect for outpatient clinics. To the benefit of owners (not so much for employees), additional revenue realized after overhead is paid greatly expands profitability. An extra ten percent of volume can mean as much as thirty percent or more profit. A clinic that has enough volume to consistently fill expanded hours definitely can be considered "niche."

The other component to profitability that can make a niche market within physical therapy is higher than average reimbursement. This could be from a concentrated, high-paying payer mix. An example is a clinic that specializes in workers compensation. It takes more effort to get and keep work comp business, but it pays better.

Clinics that have only one payer type or source can qualify as specialized, and if this is profitable then it makes it a niche. What is the best payer source in the therapy world? Perhaps it isn't a certain type of business or a certain insurance company. Contrary to common thinking, the best payment source may be the patients themselves rather than insurance companies. That's right, collecting payments directly from patients.

Cash-based therapy works for several reasons: the percentage charges compared to collections can be very high, the overall cost of collecting can be very low, the scope of practice is not limited by an insurance company's mandates, and the quality of services rendered can be very high, leading to high patient satisfaction.

Let's dive deeper.

Think you're services are better than the therapist down the street and that you deserve to be paid more? Charge whatever you want, insurance companies are only going to pay you the allowed amount that your provider contract with them stipulates. A typical physical therapy visit can easily have charges that reach $200.00 to $250.00, but the average clinic is paid $100.00 to $110.00 per visit by insurance companies. In a cash-based clinic where the patient is expected to pay, you can charge less and receive payment in full, and this payment can be more than in the insurance payment world. For example, charge $140.00, get paid $140.00.

Impressed? Let's go another step. The amount of work that is required to get the insurance company's $110.00 per visit is astounding. Therapists have to document for several reasons—payment, liability, and continuity of care. Of these, insurance company standards for payment drive documentation requirements up the most. When the notes are done, then begins the work of submitting claims to insurance companies. An easy process? Hardly. And guess what? You have to wait on insurance companies to pay you, which can take weeks or sometimes even months. Furthermore, if there is any little thing wrong with your claim submission you can be denied payment.

Once I sat across the room with a physician as he dictated. This was in the days of paper charts. He would talk into a recorder, then toss charts into a pile on the floor when he finished. "Documentation is the bane of a physician's existence," he said. It's that way for therapists, too.

This isn't a pretty picture, but it's a reality that is part and parcel with healthcare. And we haven't added in the costs of collecting yet! Having one or more employees who only submit claims and work rejections is almost a requirement. This is additional overhead that reduces profit.

In a cash-based model, there are no claims to submit, no rejections to appeal, and much less overhead is required to collect. Documentation can be focused on providing good continuity of care from one visit to the next and protecting against liability, and no extra steps are required for reimbursement. A therapist charges an overall lower amount but receives 100% of the charge. Because of this higher reimbursement, more time can be spent one-on-one with each patient. This increases patient satisfaction and overall outcomes.

It is important to note that physical therapists are not allowed to "opt out" of Medicare at this time. This means that Medicare beneficiaries cannot pay cash for PT, and those who seek to receive care from a cash-based therapist will have to be referred to a therapist who is in network with Medicare.

With all of these positives, why aren't all practices going to cash-only? The mindset of patients in the general population is that an episode of physical therapy is too expensive. In affluent communities, niche markets exist that will support cash-based therapy for athletic enhancement such as golf and tennis, and even some home health services.

As we said earlier, specialization and certification within physical therapy might not make a difference in pay in the general world, but it can make all the difference in niche markets. Having a sports certification may not bring you any more income in rural Alabama, but your specialized skills might let you market yourself to golfers in Myrtle Beach or to runners in Denver, keeping a profitable niche practice open for business.

Q&A with Aaron LeBauer

A leader in the cash-based physical therapy field is Aaron LeBauer, a physical therapist and business consultant based in North Carolina. Aaron was gracious enough to provide a lot of insight into cash-based practices. Here is our Q&A:

Question: Your "About" page tells your story of owning a cash-based massage practice before going to PT school. You started right out of school with cash-based PT in spite of your professors' disbelief! You go on to say that you definitely faced some unforeseen challenges. Will you describe one of those challenges?

Answer: "After I opened my practice I learned that I could no longer treat Medicare patients. This came out of left field and I had to learn how to deal with it. As a physical therapist in North Carolina, I am unrestricted in practice except that I cannot manipulate the spine without a physician's referral or order, and I'm not able to treat Medicare patients for a 'covered service.' I can still treat a Medicare beneficiary for 'non-covered services' such as wellness services, exercise instruction, private yoga, performance enhancement, massage therapy, and group classes. However, quite often I have to refer Medicare beneficiaries to other PT practices."

Question: Satisfied customers who are vocal about positive experiences can help a business more than any advertising campaign. We are most likely to find raving fans when we spend a lot of time with a patient. What are your thoughts on quality versus quantity for the long-term success of a therapy business?

Answer: "Quality is much more important. We have to provide high quality not only to promote ourselves, but also to promote the profession. While a larger, in-network clinic may need to see a lot of patients to meet their overhead, quality of care often suffers. In the long run, quality wins every time."

Question: How is this limited by taking insurance?

Answer: "There is a mind shift that is happening with insurance. We do not have auto insurance to pay for the maintenance on a car, like changing the oil or buying a new set of tires when they fail an inspection. We have insurance to protect against if the car is stolen or totaled. Health insurance is now the same way. The way people think of therapy services is changing, and they are beginning to become better consumers of their healthcare dollars. As therapists we have to ask ourselves what can we provide that is unique and valuable? We're not providing emergency services or services that are costing tens of thousands of dollars. The course of care may cost $2,000, and that's usually deductible. It's a mindset shift that is happening. Once we get to that point, it's kind of like there really is no difference. The only difference is that I don't do the administrative processing of the claim for the patients. I provide them with the information and they do it themselves."

Question: Let me make sure I understand this right. I'm not going to ask what your charges are, but let's use this as an example. You charge $150 per visit and the patient has to pay cash but it goes against their deductible and they get one-on-one treatment. If they go to another insurance-based clinic, their charges for a visit might reach $250, and since it goes against their deductible they have to pay it, right?

Answer: "Exactly! I think the problem is people don't understand that yet because the bill usually shows up after therapy is completed. They process everything through the insurance company and then the patient gets a bill for $2,000."

Question: Do you think cash-based models will work everywhere, or is it going to be more successful in more affluent areas?

Answer: "Yes. It works anywhere. Even in towns of 3,000 people, but not in the way you position it in New York City. If you can provide a service that is not readily available or is higher quality than what people get elsewhere it is going to work. It just depends on mindset and how you position it.

Full interview with Aaron LeBauer is available here

http://bit.ly/1ZZKsK6

Niche Markets "Raise the Ceiling" Scores:

Required Overhead — Neutral. This can depend on the type of business. A sports medicine clinic with thousands of square feet of floor space for exercise equipment will have much higher overhead than a business that provides home care. A cash-based clinic will require less overhead for collections.

Financial Risk — Neutral. The amount of overhead as well as the possibility of competition determine the financial risks.

Revenue Opportunity — Favorable. By definition, niche markets are profitable. Once I heard an orthopedic surgeon quip that he specialized in "high liability, low reimbursement" cases. This could happen, of course, but generally speaking, niche therapy practices provide highly reimbursed procedures or have concentrated and high paying payer mixes, or both.

Slowlane vs. Fastlane — Slowlane, with potential to move toward Fastlane. If a business owner is able to expand the clinic to have multiple therapists and multiple locations, then this is moving toward Fastlane.

"Time for Money" vs. Passive Income — Unfavorable. Niche markets do not change the time for money issue common to physical therapy.

Scale — Unfavorable to Favorable. There's still just one of you. And niche markets are, by nature, not everywhere. This makes scaling even more difficult. If the market is strong enough for a clinic to expand its operations, then this can be favorable to business owners, which can be a good thing *if you are the owner*.

Time Frame To Success — Unfavorable. Depending on the success of marketing, it can take months to fill up a therapist's schedule. Factor in the necessary overhead involved to run the business and it may take many more months to reach profitability.

Long-Term Potential for Increased Income — Favorable. Many elements play into this: how well the business is run, how well overhead is managed, how many patients are seen each week. Niche practices are desirable because of their profitability. Just keep in mind that it doesn't happen overnight.

Potential for Sale at Exit — Neutral. Is the business in a good location, with a strong payer mix, solid leadership beneath the owner(s), with low competition and a history of profitability? These things are more likely with niche practices, which could raise the potential for an acquisition. If the business is marginal, and especially if the owner is the main therapist, this potential is much lower.

	Niche Markets
Required Overhead	Neutral
Financial Risks	Neutral
Revenue Opportunity	Favorable
Slowlane vs. Fastlane	Slowlane
"Time for Money" vs. Passive Income	Unfavorable
Scale	Neutral
Time Frame to Success	Unfavorable
Longterm Potential for Increased Income	Favorable
Potential for Sale at Exit	Neutral

Solo Clinics

It may come as a surprise to you when we have talked so much about the problems in the insurance payment world that an entire section would be included that promotes the idea of solo clinics. And by that phrase I mean outpatient practices that employee only one person: the physical therapist owner.

How can this work, and why does this have a place here?

Just in the past month there have been two different announcements of major physical therapy companies merging together. This is all driven by businesses decreasing reimbursement and increasing overhead. The goal is simple. Large corporations are able to drive down costs with economies of scale, and expanding volume increases profits for owners and investors.

If many private practice clinics can't afford to operate and they sell out to the mid-level players, and if the mid-level players sell out, and if the large corporations sell out as well, how can solo clinicians have any hope of making it independently?

The simple answer is to keep overhead extremely low and to not divide the pie with anyone.

Let's expound on that a little.

Most healthcare businesses have two major expense items: their facilities and equipment together are one, and their staff is the other.

Physical therapy, like other fields in healthcare, can fill a large space with tens of thousands of dollars worth of equipment. Therapy gyms are eye candy, and are showcased by hospitals with floor-to-ceiling windows and twenty-four hour lighting so passersby can see the magic place inside. While very alluring and certainly a good marketing tactic, top physical therapists do not always need this much equipment. In fact, it is possible—and from a business standpoint, *advisable*—to not have much equipment at all.

It is common understanding among therapists that patients who regularly perform their home exercise program as instructed will have better outcomes than those who do not. Compliance is the critical factor in this, so it is essential that patients understand what to do and how to perform exercises correctly. To build this understanding and reinforce the need for compliance, therapists can utilize clinic time toward teaching and advancing home exercise programs. The only equipment necessary for this are tools that either a patient already has in their homes, or tools that can be sold or given to the patient at a reasonable cost.

Taking this concept to an extreme liberates clinics from large, costly gyms and the expense of multiple pieces of expensive equipment. Patients who receive extensive training for home exercise will appreciate the coaching from their therapist more than those who use exercise equipment without a lot of personal direction. For this to happen, all that is required is a therapist with good skills, a mat or table, and a few inexpensive home exercise tools. What's more, patients respond to hands-on care and one-on-one training in a more positive way than they do using exercise equipment.

I asked Aaron LeBauer, who has a "low overhead practice" if his patients were skeptical of his skills because he didn't have a therapy gym full of equipment. Here's his response:

"If they are [skeptical] I haven't heard about it. Usually what I hear is that people appreciate the one-on-one time. They will tell me that they went to another therapy clinic and they were put on machines, being left alone and doing exercises that they could do at home or at their gym. Our patients appreciate the private, quiet, and focused attention and experience at our practice much better."

This combination of patient preferences and low costs creates an opportunity for physical therapists. A practice where extensive one-on-one time is provided will be well received by patients and develop a strong reputation within a community.

In looking at facilities as a major expense, the location of the facility is critical. A balance has to be struck between finding a reputable part of the community and securing low rent. A solid reputation will bring patients off of the beaten path, but not into an undesirable area. Remember that a clinic's patients come largely from the surrounding community, and affluent areas will have strongest payer mixes.

For a solo practice to be successful, overhead has to be tightly controlled. The other large expense for all healthcare businesses is staff. Utilizing lower hourly wage personnel to perform unskilled tasks to free up knowledge workers to perform professional tasks has been the mantra in healthcare for decades. When we get this out of order, bad things happen to business finances. A joke among doctors who don't like electronic medical records is that M.D. stands for "making decisions," not "making data." It's that way in the PT world, too.

Large therapy clinics have support personnel to help with clinic cleaning, laundry, restocking supply rooms, registration, telephone calls and many, many other essential duties. These tasks are part of healthcare and they don't go away, and it isn't efficient for a PT to be sweeping the floor. Sometimes support staff are very productive, but sometimes there isn't enough work to keep them busy. Large organizations can afford this inefficiency. Small practices should look for every possible means to keep costs low.

Outsourcing can be a solution. Cleaning, laundry, billing, even telephone support can all be contracted to outside vendors. There is a cost with this, of course. Established businesses that consider reducing overhead in this way will have to evaluate the costs of outsourcing in their area versus the cost of keeping employees, and they will have to decide if the savings is worth parting with long-term staff. New businesses, especially small, solo-practices, have the advantage because the volume of unskilled tasks is relatively low, and the total cost of all outsourcing can be less than hiring a full-time support person.

It takes effort to find outsourcing companies that can meet the needs of therapists, but it can be cheaper to outsource than to hire support staff. For the goal of keeping overhead as low as possible, this is essential.

The lowest cost resource that is available to any healthcare provider is the patient. Can the patient enter their information directly into a record system? Computerized registration and payment systems shift burden away from support staff, often eliminating the need for employees. Some electronic medical record systems have these tools built in, while others allow third-party add-ons that support these functions. These tools aren't free, but they can be cheaper than hiring staff.

A therapist can operate a solo practice with little to no office staff if support needs are outsourced to human and software companies. These contracts should be service-based, so that monthly expenses will rise and fall with clinic volume.

Combining a philosophy of hands-on care, minimizing total clinic square footage and capital expenditures on equipment, and reducing support staff to a minimum can provide solo practitioners an optimal overhead percentage from which to operate a business. Combine a solo practice with a niche market and this can help even more.

The information above is based on my business experience managing larger practices. Operating a solo practice hasn't been my journey, but many therapists make their living with this type of business.

Q&A with Jarod Carter, DPT

A leader in the solo practice field is Jarod Carter, a physical therapist in Austin, Texas. His practice, Carter Physiotherapy, has been in a solo practice business since 2010. Only recently has he added another physical therapist.

Jarod invited me on his podcast to do a reverse interview. It was great fun! I asked him to describe the moment when he realized that not only was he going to open a solo practice but that it would also be a cash-based clinic. Here's his response:

"In the beginning, I got into a situation where the private practice I was working with wanted to change my payment arrangement in a way that I really couldn't accept. I decided it was best I move on.

For a while I was a private physical therapist for a relatively wealthy couple that needed a lot of treatment. I did that about a year, eight years ago. As that was happening, I tried to figure what my next step was going to be. I wasn't really pumped about going back to work for anyone.

When I was traveling with that couple after I'd left my previous job, I started to have some patients who sought me out and found me on LinkedIn and Twitter. I realized that I had a handful of people that were at the moment really wanting to continue treatment with me. And so I said, 'You know what?...I'm just gonna go for it.'

The reason I chose cash-based is because I worked in insurance-based practices, and I worked in cash-based practice. I saw the trends of declining reimbursements and the headaches dealing with insurance. I decided to start cash pay and figured, if worse comes to worse, I can just convert and start to take insurance."

While cash-based, and for several years a solo practice, Jarod does have a clinic. This not the only model available to PTs.

Full interview with Jarod Carter is available here.

http://bit.ly/1UpUPFl

Q&A with Karen Litzy, DPT

Karen Litzy, host of the Healthy, Wealthy and Smart podcast about physical therapy, is a solo physical therapist in New York City. Her practice is unique because she doesn't have a clinic! She performs outpatient therapy in her patients' homes or at their work places.

Karen has websites for her podcast and her practice. She also spoke with me for this book— her story is really incredible!

Question: Your "About Karen" page describes how you "became overwhelmed with requests" to treat patients in their homes of offices. How did you find yourself in this position?

Answer: "When I first moved to New York City, I worked in a very large gym…I saw a lot of the personal trainers working with their clients at home or their home gyms or businesses. I thought, 'Why can't I do that?'

When you live in a place like New York City where people are busy and your days are packed it's just nice to have someone come to you. That way you don't have to leave work. I go to patients' offices. A lot of the offices have gyms in them. I had one patient say that he did go to an outpatient clinic and he remarked, 'You know, to get to a clinic and do therapy takes two hours out of my day. I manage over a billion dollars a day, I don't have time to be out of the office for a few hours.'

And so, it's just that the convenience factor is so high for people. That's why people kept asking for me to see people in the home."

Question: Having low overhead is incredibly important to any business. Will you describe the overhead in your practice?

Answer: "The main overhead in my practice is very, very low. I've got my Metrocard, which in New York it's how you get on the subway and the buses. I've got the upkeep of websites and things like that, which is not terribly expensive. Oh, and taxis. And WebPT. If I buy any equipment like a biofeedback machine and theraband. Continuing education is a big chunk of change, percentage wise, but compared to a typical business it's not."

Question: Word of mouth is without question the best form of advertising. Second to this is for people to already have a relationship with you, to feel like they know you already. Corporations spend millions and billions each year on branding just for this purpose. Your path for branding is very unique: podcasting. How has this helped your therapy business?

Answer: "The radio show is a podcast. It is mainly for therapists and has actually helped with my business because I get therapists from around the world referring patients to me. I've had people from South Africa and Europe refer patients to me because they know me.

I will refer some patients to a podcast episode that might be pertinent to them. I do a lot of episodes on pain because a lot of my clients' problems are chronic pain. And I do curate tons of episodes on pain. For instance, when I'm interviewing an expert on pain and think that this is going to be something that's really going to benefit one of my patients, I will direct them to it.

Because, I've had people say to me, well, you're not really an entrepreneur.

'Well, you're not really an entrepreneur because it's just you.' When you have a business and you're in business and have all the risks of business are there... And I was, like, I'm pretty sure I'm an entrepreneur. I mean, I own my own business. I have a tax ID number. I pay a lot of taxes. They would say, 'you're not scalable. You're really not an entrepreneur.' But I think it's total, total crap by the way. The podcast is pretty scalable. I do get 10,000 downloads a month and it is downloaded in 100 different countries."

Full interview with Karen Litzy is available here

http://bit.ly/1XxepTN

Before we move into the scores of this section, here are a few points that are part of successful solo practices:

- Positioning yourself in rural areas where there is little competition can make success easier, but it can also mean a payer mix with lower paying insurances.

- Positioning yourself in urban areas increases opportunities for concierge-type services where you can tailor your practice to meet the needs of patients who are willing to pay you a very high rate.

- Keep costs as low as possible. Most therapy clinics are full of equipment. The only equipment a therapist really needs to have is what a patient will have at home. Teach the patient to do a home program and be hands-on with the patient more. Less equipment, less equipment overhead.

- The less equipment there is, the less equipment overhead you'll have and the less space you'll need for it. Keep space and rent to a minimum.

- Utilize inexpensive software and pay for the software company to do your billing. This will eliminate the need for additional staff. Several software packages are available for this, and prices usually start around $50 per month depending on which services are needed.

- Cater to special interest groups, especially those that are cash-based.

Solo Clinics "Raise the Ceiling" Scores:

Required Overhead — Favorable. Solo therapists can position themselves for financial success by keeping overhead as low as possible. Hands-on care is perceived as higher quality than exercising on machines. It doesn't take much space for a solo therapist to run an outpatient clinic if there isn't much equipment. Keep electronic systems and phone systems to a minimum. Automate as many processes as possible, and outsource to avoid paying for support staff. If possible, eliminate the need to bill insurance companies and take cash only. Look for guerrilla marketing tactics that are low-cost but still generate a buzz.

Financial Risk — Neutral to Favorable. Because overhead can be kept low, there is less at risk.

Revenue Opportunity — Neutral. This depends on the community where the clinic is located and its payer source. Niche-based practices or those with a strong payer mix will have a more favorable opportunity. The great advantage is that the therapist can keep profits rather than these going to business shareholders. This alone does not guarantee success or high income, as the business still has to be run well, with efficiency and consistency.

Slowlane vs. Fastlane — Slowlane. If you are the only employee of the business, then the business does not run without your presence.

"Time for Money" vs. Passive Income —Highly Unfavorable. A solo clinic operates under the time for money exchange. With cash flow being interrupted if the therapist owner takes a vacation, in regard to passive income this model is less favorable than being an employee of another business and having earned time off.

Scale — Unfavorable to Favorable. There's just one of you. Your reach will be limited by your community and by your time. If the market is strong enough for you to add therapists and expand operations, then this can be favorable.

Time Frame To Success — Unfavorable to Neutral. Depending on the success of marketing, it can take months to fill up a therapist's schedule. Factor in the necessary overhead involved to run the business and it may take many more months to reach profitability.

Long-Term Potential for Increased Income — Neutral to Favorable. Many elements play into this: how well the business is run, how well overhead is managed, how many patients are seen each week, how strong the payer source is, and how strong the referral sources are. Solo practices are desirable because therapists can work for themselves and develop their own brand. Not all situations or environments will produce optimal results.

Potential for Sale at Exit — Highly Unfavorable. The nature of a solo clinic is that the owner is the main therapist. Even though therapists can minimize overhead, have complete control of their business, and enjoy strong incomes, unless additional therapists or other revenue streams are added to the practice that will attract buyers, an acquisition with a high multiple is not likely.

	Solo Clinics
Required Overhead	Favorable
Financial Risks	Neutral
Revenue Opportunity	Neutral
Slowlane vs. Fastlane	Slowlane
"Time for Money" vs. Passive Income	Highly Unfavorable
Scale	Neutral
Time Frame to Success	Unfavorable
Longterm Potential for Increased Income	Neutral
Potential for Sale at Exit	Unfavorable

Minority Ownership Clinic

Some large corporations recruit and retain therapists by offering minority ownership in individual clinics. Therapists have to invest money at the start, perhaps ten to twenty-five percent of initial costs, which can be $10,000 to $25,000. Though they don't have a controlling interest in the business, they still reap the rewards of strong financial performance.

For therapists, this arrangement provides many stabilities: expanded startup capital with decreased risk, corporate training, corporate marketing, compliance programs, recruiting help, strategic planning and leadership, and expanded income. For companies, therapists with "skin in the game" are very loyal and committed to the financial performance of clinics. This is a win-win scenario.

Therapists who are owners in a practice work for a regular salary, but are able to participate in quarterly distributions. It is possible for therapists to have minority ownership in multiple practices, receiving income from them all.

Minority Ownership Clinic "Raise the Ceiling" Scores:

Required Overhead — Unfavorable. This can depend on the type of business, but most general outpatient PT practices have large footprints and expensive exercise equipment. This will be more expensive if the facility is in a prime location. Even though minority owners have assistance covering expenses, overhead is a major item in the most basic business formulas and cannot be neglected. Managing overhead will be necessary to realize a quarterly distribution.

Financial Risks — Unfavorable to Neutral. The more spent on overhead, the more is at risk. The better the location, the more likely it is that a competitor will come in and take away market share. For minority owners, risks are offset by partnership with the larger organization.

Revenue Opportunity — Neutral to Favorable. Physical therapy is a profitable business. With a corporate guidance, it is easier to operate with margins that are tight.

Slowlane vs. Fastlane — Slowlane, with potential to move toward Fastlane. If a minority owner is able to expand the clinic to have multiple therapists and multiple locations, then this is moving toward Fastlane.

"Time for Money" vs. Passive Income — Unfavorable. Outpatient private practices do not change the time for money issue common to physical therapy.

Scale — Unfavorable to Favorable. Therapy businesses are complicated. If you are working 'in' the business as well as the person who works "on" the business, then growing can be difficult. If the market is strong enough for a clinic to expand its operations, then this can be favorable.

Time Frame To Success — Neutral. Depending on the success of marketing, it can take months to fill up a therapist's schedule. Factor in the necessary overhead involved to run the business and it may take many more months to reach profitability. This can be easier when partnered with a large corporation that is accustomed to starting new clinics.

Longterm Potential for Increased Income — Favorable. If outside and uncontrollable forces do not negatively impact the business, outpatient private practices can be quite profitable.

Many elements play into this: how well the business is run, how well overhead is managed, how many patients are seen each week, the number of locations. Large companies will help guide minority owners to reach optimal performance.

Potential for Sale at Exit — Favorable. It is likely that terms of sale of minority ownership will be written into the initial contracts with a pre-defined multiple. Minority owners are not selling the entire company, only their portion, so expect these multiples to be on the lower end of the spectrum.

	Minority Ownership Clinics
Required Overhead	Unfavorable
Financial Risks	Unfavorable
Revenue Opportunity	Neutral
Slowlane vs. Fastlane	Slowlane
"Time for Money" vs. Passive Income	Unfavorable
Scale	Neutral
Time Frame to Success	Neutral
Longterm Potential for Increased Income	Favorable
Potential for Sale at Exit	Favorable

Contract Therapy Services

Managing all of the line items in a business is difficult. For a lot of therapists, the very idea of looking at a profit and loss statement causes as much anxiety as going to math class. Fortunately, there is a business structure that minimizes some of the business risks and limits the scope of business to just providing therapists.

Enter Contract Therapy Services.

Fortunately, the demand for therapists is high. This is because government regulations require that children with special needs receive care, and patients admitted to long-term care facilities and home health agencies receive evaluations within twenty-four hours of their admission. Therapy businesses of all types have regular turnover as well as maternity and paternity leaves and often need fill-in staff to help cover their volume. Rural areas are less attractive to young professionals, and often nursing home administrators in these locations are not skilled at hiring therapists. This vacuum creates a space for large and small business to provide therapists to healthcare entities that would rather contract this job to someone else then put continual effort into maintaining a therapist staff.

Just what types of opportunities are out there? Here are a few examples that I have witnessed in my career:

- A therapist contracts to provide therapy services by herself to a school system. In time, she hires another person to help with the caseload. She earns a reputation for doing good work and being dependable. Other school systems struggle finding therapists and they call on her. She brings on more help and expands her operation. This happens time and again, and her business grows to several school systems in multiple counties.

- A therapist signs on to do PRN work for Company A in the long-term care industry. He learns the ropes of the business while working, and he sees an opportunity when very rural areas are hard to serve, even for Company A. He knows a few therapists who are willing to help him, and he creates a company of his own to go into these areas to provide therapy services. At first, he sub-contracts with Company A. His success comes because of his connection with therapists, not because of his experience. (For rural areas, having a therapist—even one with limited experience—is better than not having one.) His company grows to service several nursing homes, eventually stealing facilities that initially had contracts with Company A.

- A therapist is asked to provide contract therapy services for a startup home health company. This is a new venture, but she is able to put together a small team of friends and colleagues to meet the need. With a company established, other business opportunities present themselves, including school systems, other home health agencies, and rural hospitals. In time, the initial home health agency goes under, but by then the new therapy company is able to survive on the strength of other business. A larger hospital provides a lucrative contract for this company to provide both inpatient and outpatient services.

- A nursing home owner decides he wants to offer therapy services not only at his facility, but at other facilities in the surrounding area, as well. A small therapy company is formed. They quickly grow to provide services at five facilities. Over the course of seventeen years the company grows to service over thirty facilities and expands their service lines into outpatient and home health.

- In similar fashion to the last case, a therapist with a therapy company is asked to provide outpatient services in an orthopedic physician practice with an arrangement where the physicians are part owners. While controversial, this proves to be legal and profitable. Taking the opportunity, the therapist grows this company from one clinic in one location to having over two hundred and fifty therapists in over seventy clinics all across the country in under ten years.

As these examples illustrate, contract therapy can create a very strong business. To be successful, a strong network of therapists is needed. Recruiting therapists will be a regular activity, as will educating new staff on employment policies and documentation requirements. There are many opportunities for contract companies if internal development can keep up with growth. A therapist owner will need support staff and additional managers as volume increases. Long-term success is dependent on the quality of the management team that is built more than the number of contracts. Complexity increases exponentially.

In order to grow, it will also be necessary to negotiate payment rates that are favorable for all parties. This requires understanding the reimbursement model for facilities to set rates appropriately. Some markets are competitive. Bidding wars with other contract companies can be very disruptive to overall profits. A pricing "race to the bottom" can be detrimental. It is necessary to provide quality above your premium in order to keep business and to not have to renegotiate at the end of every contract term.

Q&A with Myra Bolton Scott, OT

Myra Bolton Scott has been the President of Champion, Partners in Rehab, a contract therapy company, since the company began seventeen years ago. She took a few minutes out of her busy routine to speak with me for this book. Here are a few questions and answers from our conversation:

Question: Your success has come in the long-term care contract therapy service business. Did you choose this niche because of its advantages, or were you at the right place at the right time with the right skills and the right desires for the opportunity? In other words, did you choose the path, or did the path choose you? How much of a difference does this make in the success a therapist can have?

Answer: "I've never wanted to do long-term care. That was not my choice. When I got out of school, actually, my love was pediatrics. I thought that was what I wanted to do. I did one of my clinicals at Children's Hospital and one of the things that I realized pretty quickly is that I was a little too tender-hearted for it. It was rewarding, but I was personally a wreck because I took it home with me every single day.

Long-term care was not what I had set out to do. Then, I had an opportunity to do some PRN work in long term-care setting with my grandmother.

My grandmother had been in a nursing home and it just so happened that back in that time, therapy was just getting going in the school nursing settings... [Long-term care is] not something that I even thought I wanted to do, but once I was working in that setting, I didn't want to leave it.

As far as choosing the path or the path choosing you, I think a lot of it has to do with being at the right place at the right time. But I also think that people can make things happen even when what's happening around them is not the most ideal thing."

Question: It's much easier to sell than it is to build and maintain long-term business relationships. Contract companies that divert energy to growth away from existing customers risk losing them. Your philosophy has always to grow within the state. How did you come to have this belief, and how has it served you as Champion matured?

Answer: "I always felt—and I still feel this way—that whatever growth you have needs to be managed growth and not growth for growth's sake. I never felt that we were at the point that I could give my full attention to growth outside of the state, and there were still too many opportunities close to home. You look at what the low-hanging fruit is like. If there's still opportunity close to home, if we're still growing, if we're choosing goals with resources that we have without adding that factor of distance…I'm certainly not against growing outside of the state, and I feel that at some point we will.

We have walked away from some opportunities because I just felt our reputation was on the line. If we were losing business on one end because we're gaining on the other, where is the sense in that? The energy that you put in to grow a new business, wow, it takes a lot to get something up and running, get your folks loyal and dedicated, and having the will to put it all spinning. Why on earth would you walk away from it to do that all over again if you can't keep your eye on what you've got going already?"

Question: It's one thing to want to build a company, it's another to navigate the challenges of business and changes in health care year after year. This isn't something that they teach you in therapy school! What skills and methods and resources have served you best in your journey, and how did you learn about them?

Answer: "You know, one of the things I said when we started Champion was that any decisions we made I want us to always take into account how it affected the patients, how it affected our customers, how it affected the employees, was it ethical and legal, and was it financially sound.

Even in the crazy, crazy world of healthcare and with all the reimbursement challenges and all the government rules and regulations, I can honestly say that with every major decision, I have always tried to look at these things: how is it going to affect our patients, how is it going to affect our employees, our customers, is it legal and is it financially sound.

And I think with those five guiding principles, that's why we've been successful. That's our compass. Most every major decision, we put through the test of those five things and really define those as the five driving forces of the company. It's not always clear cut and easy, but I think having defined those guiding factors has made all the difference in the world."

Full interview with Myra Bolton Scott is available here

http://bit.ly/1PAsrw3

Q&A with Tom Pennington, PT

Tom Pennington is the co-founder of Physician Rehab Solutions. During his life he has owned three therapy companies, the previous two being DiversiCare Rehab Group, a regional rehab company, and Integrity Rehab Group, the largest physical-based rehab company in the nation. Tom graciously agreed to answer a few questions for this book.

Question: How did you learn to build businesses?

Answer: "I had no formal training in learning to build a business. I knew that when I was in physical therapy school, for better or worse, I wanted to control my own destiny and be my own master, and didn't want to be subjected to hospital bureaucracy or a company or ownership where I became a pawn in whatever decisions they made, good or bad. That was not necessarily reflective of a success that I would have in my local operation.

I graduated from PT school in 1983. I had no formal management or business classes, but I did have a very good instructor that was world-class in his administrative capacities. His project of helping us design and budget for our own hospital department was a first step in recognizing some of the financial ramifications that existed in what I thought was the coolest profession in the world—physical therapy. I really learned to build the business in a very rudimentary fashion of a Nike saying, "Just do it," and was fortunate enough in the process that I did not go bankrupt.

I was also fortunate enough to bring on a tremendously talented individual who had a strong grasp of the management and finances of the business, and he quickly assessed our company from a financial vantage point and made strong recommendations. He gave us an opportunity to work smarter, not harder, and it was a tremendous relief that I could focus on the clinical and have someone of equal knowledge and expertise on the financial.

But the bottom line to me is ... that it is best to recognize your strengths and put your emphasis and attention into that, and surround yourself with people that have strengths that compensate for your weaknesses. I have been blessed to have been able to have people of integrity and talent around me for the last 20 years, which have compensated for my lack of talent in respective areas of administration, finance, clinical development, human resources, and marketing."

Question: In recent years you have been in the outpatient contract therapy service business. Did you choose this niche because of its advantages or were you at the right place at the right time with the right skills and the right desires for the opportunity? In other words, did you choose the path, or did the path choose you?

Answer: "We have been in the outpatient contracting service by design. My partner and I were challenged several years ago [by a consultant] ... to be the best we could be at one particular service line. We looked at the state of Medicare and Medicaid and where our profession was going with trying to provide the best outcomes in the lowest cost setting, we decided to emphasize and champion one of our existing service lines, which was private practice which contracted, staffed, and managed outpatient clinics in physician settings. Physicians were expanding their services, at many times doing it without therapists being involved by using athletic trainers, exercise physiologists, etc. but to the general public looking like physical therapist services. When we looked at all the models from our freestanding outpatient clinics to hospital outpatient to our physician outpatient models, it was not even close on what setting provided the best outcomes at the fewest visits and at the lowest costs coupled with the highest patient satisfaction and physician satisfaction.

So it was very strategic that we looked at [contract] outpatient therapy services, because it was in the best interest of all stakeholders—the patients, the payer sources, our therapists for professional growth opportunities, and our physician referral sources. So we were intentional about choosing the path, but we were very fortunate that we were already on this path and several others to be able to judge the quality of the path and where this path would lead."

Question: How much of a difference does finding the right path make in the success a therapist can have?

Answer: "I think choosing the right path does make a significant difference in the success that a therapist can have, but I think there are many paths to success. Obviously, you don't want to choose a path in which you go against your ability, so that needs to be ruled out immediately. With that said, I don't think it was as much the path that you take, but it's the creativity, the originality, and the hard work and passion that you provide while working on whatever path you are going down. Like any path, if you run into large trees or boulders, you will probably have to pick a new path. Hence, know your path but have a level of flexibility as obstacles arise. I see a lot of therapists and a lot of companies that are stuck in a paradigm of the past and stubbornly refuse to change until it's too late. Isn't that always the key—to have passion and stubbornness but not to the point of failure?"

Question: Is it easier for a contract company to add new business or to maintain existing relationships? Which works out better for the long-term health of the organization?

Answer: "I don't think it is normally one or the other in regard to adding new business or maintaining existing relationships. I think that both bear equal importance in the long-term health of the organization. On a contract basis, you certainly want to work toward sustaining value to be able to renew existing clients and contracts, but at the same time realize that a certain amount of contracts will not be renewed for various reasons, and that growth will have to add to offset any potential loss of business in the future. So I place equal importance on existing business and adding additional business at the same time."

Full interview with Tom Pennington is available here

http://bit.ly/1Y2aOOb

Contract Therapy Services "Raise the Ceiling" Scores:

Required Overhead — Favorable. Operational overhead can be kept extremely low in contract businesses as the employed therapists are the face of the organization, not the home office. Many companies repurpose inexpensive residential homes as office space. Remodeling and updated furniture are spared to keep overhead as low as possible. Staff costs, however, are not inexpensive. PRN rates are high for therapists, and contract services are often required in areas of therapy that pay higher salaries. Great care will be needed to control every component of overhead as occasionally it may be necessary to pay a therapist a ridiculous rate in order to meet contract requirements with a facility.

Financial Risks — Favorable. The burden here becomes having sufficient cash flow to make payroll two or three times each month. Be careful to structure your contracts in a way that covers all costs in as close to real-time as possible.

Revenue Opportunity — Favorable to Highly Favorable. There are several methods of setting rates: sometimes a percentage of profit is used, sometimes a percentage of reimbursement, and sometimes companies are paid an hourly rate. Rural hospitals and nursing homes are required to provide therapy services. In some locations where therapists are very difficult to find, facilities will take a loss on therapy services in order to be in compliance with government regulations. These situations can be very profitable for therapy companies.

Slowlane vs. Fastlane — Fastlane. The contract therapy arena provides one of the key components that makes a fastlane business: SCALE. Strong business models and strong management teams can quickly expand their reach to multiple facilities. Their only limiting factor will be their ability to develop as quickly as they can grow while keeping their current customers satisfied with the value they provide. Adding new business is only growth if old contracts are maintained. Wisdom in leadership is needed here. I have watched rehab companies grow too fast and lose initial contracts. It can be just as profitable with much less effort to stay small while delivering high value than growing too fast and losing business in the process.

"Time for Money" vs. Passive Income — Neutral. Physical therapy is a "time for money" business, and that never changes. As contract service businesses grow, owners and leaders shift their duties. It can happen that management structure is strong enough for an owner to completely step out of day-to-day operations, but usually this doesn't happen fully until the business is sold. Facilities are the customer, and if the customer isn't happy senior managers and owners have to drop everything to help fix problems. This potential increases with the size of a company.

Scale — Highly Favorable. Contract Service businesses are definitely fastlane.

Time Frame To Success — Favorable. Set your rates and hire your staff and go to work. There will be ups and downs, and you have to run your business efficiently. It can be possible to have positive cash flow in just a few months.

Long-Term Potential for Increased Income — Highly Favorable. Once business foundations are built, contract service businesses can scale. Limits on this are set either by market forces or by leadership decisions.

Potential for Sale at Exit — Highly Favorable. With a history of profitability, a strong leadership team, multiple service locations, and strong contractual agreements acquisition is highly favorable.

	Contract Therapy Services
Required Overhead	Favorable
Financial Risks	Favorable
Revenue Opportunity	Favorable
Slowlane vs. Fastlane	Fastlane
"Time for Money" vs. Passive Income	Neutral
Scale	Highly Favorable
Time Frame to Success	Highly Favorable
Longterm Potential for Increased Income	Highly Favorable
Potential for Sale at Exit	Highly Favorable

****

Reminder — *to overcome fear, you have to see yourself as being a person who can overcome whatever it is that makes you afraid. You have to see yourself as a person worthy of success. Daily habits that focus on your confidence as well as your knowledge and your connections will help you develop into a person who will accomplish your goals.*

****

Chapter 14

Opportunities in Supporting PT Industries

*"Instead of thinking outside the box, get rid of the box." —
Deepak Chopra*

Just joining us? I'm sure a lot of people will just skip straight to this chapter.

So far we've covered the abundant job opportunities that are available in the PT field, we've talked about how therapists can see significant pay raises with job changes during the first decade of their careers before hitting an income ceiling, and we've looked at several paths to business ownership within physical therapy, scoring each one for its individual business strengths and weaknesses.

If you are picking up the book here, go back to the section titled "Second Recertification: Slowlane and Fastlane" before you continue reading. There are some concepts there that you won't want to miss!

Ready to move ahead? Ready to learn how to raise the ceiling in non-typical ways?

First, a warning.

The information in this section is not a way to make more money at your current job. It's not even a sure method to make more money, period. You can easily lose money. Lots of it. Business has risks. Plenty of therapists close down therapy businesses each year. Even more entrepreneurs close shops and stores and end product lines when they don't work out. Enter at your own peril.

I'll say it again: it is entirely possible to lose money on any of the ideas that follow. If you're going to lose money, don't lose borrowed money. No risk, no reward? Sure, but don't take stupid risks. Seek advice from professionals and read everything you can get your hands on before starting out. Therapists have little or no business training, after all. Get help. Get advice.

Now, with that disclaimer behind us, remember:

NO RISK, NO REWARD

NOTHING VENTURED, NOTHING GAINED

And one more warning.

If you continue to do the same thing you have always done, it's almost guaranteed that you will get the same thing you have always gotten.

Getting out of your comfort zone isn't for the faint of heart. Business owners all take risks, and you will have to as well. Trust your ability to acquire new skills—you made it through therapy school after all, right? Learn everywhere. Read everything you can get your hands on. Listen to podcasts and audiobooks on business. Work hard and develop yourself and your confidence. Don't be afraid to lose sight of shore, but remember that you are going to be in deep water. You'll need some good maps and good instruments, and you might need to hire a good sailor now and then.

> "Life in the fastlane, surely make you lose your mind." -The Eagles

Did you notice a trend as we made our way through the last section? Every business type was directly involved in physical therapy practice. Most are Slowlane. Only the business types that scale have Fastlane tendencies.

Is there money to be made in the traditional physical therapy model? Absolutely. Physical therapy gives you a good-sized shovel to dig with right in your own backyard. Many therapists who have their own businesses enjoy tremendous incomes. Building your own standard PT business can be fantastically rewarding and profitable. It can also be a job.

Let's review the definition of Fastlane. This term comes from MJ DeMarco's book, *The Millionaire Fastlane.* According to DeMarco, the Fastlane uses controllable, unlimited leverage for growth. Therapists have limited leverage because they trade time for money. Scaling success to achieve a one hundred or one thousand percent return in traditional models means growing a business to have hundreds of employees. This can be done, and many have done it, but it requires great overhead and many years of effort. In a Fastlane business, a high level of wealth can be achieved with five to ten years of focused and accountable work. The Fastlane doesn't avoid work, but it focuses on building systems that do the work, optimizing and automating relentlessly. It shifts focus from being a person who buys late-night infomercial products to a person producing and selling them, from being a worker *in* the business to being a person who works *on* the business, from being a person who buys a franchise to being the person who sells franchises.

As we move forward we will be talking about types of businesses that all physical therapists are qualified to start but that do not involve providing care. Instead, they provide educational and service products within the physical therapy industry. These businesses are governed by the rules of the free market, and are not limited by the number of square feet in the clinic or the size of their community, but by the size of target audiences and the ease or difficulty of getting them to buy.

The power of the Internet gives us incredible reach around the world to coordinate with freelancers, designers, producers, distributors, and most importantly, buyers. Every bit of this happens every day within the physical therapy world. There are millions of dollars spent on books and seminars and products each year. It's already there, a supporting industry for the profession of physical therapy that can be 100% Fastlane. And every bit of it is within reach of a physical therapist with desire and some business savvy.

As the old saying goes, "Rome wasn't built in a day." Neither are therapy businesses. Not the ones that take care of patients, not the ones that don't. The scale of the Internet lets therapists reach the masses with almost no limit. What is necessary is the know-how to go from desire to idea to action to a viable business to success. There can be a tremendous learning curve, but because of the nature of this type of business, progress that is slow at the start can grow exponentially when the ingredients are mixed just right. With no "time for money" exchange, there are ways to leverage your knowledge and experience that can bring a tremendous return.

In this section, we'll look at PT product businesses that include clinical education, PT business education, PT business consultation, different types of software, and newly invented products related to clinical care. For each we'll discuss their underpinnings and growth strategies; we'll look at components to their business structures and their scores for Slowlane vs. Fastlane, etc. like we did in the last section; and we'll highlight some business owners and let them speak for themselves about entrepreneurialism.

Educational Products

Part and parcel with physical therapy is physical therapy education. We honor the gurus of the field, the university teachers and professors that inspired us, and the movement-leading experts whose work is found in professional journals and is foundational to certifications. There is always something new to learn, and those who have knowledge attract followers.

As the decades pass, the household names of PT change. Scully and Barnes and Hoppenfield have given way to Paris and Wise and Wilk, to Kisner and Colby. New educators will rise on the scene and pen the textbooks and be the thought leaders within physical therapy in the future.

The education industry is struggling to keep its identity in the digital age. Textbook companies have always made their money through physical book sales with high profit margins. There is less overhead in a digital book, but also less profit, and students are used to getting high-quality, interactive products for reasonable prices. Smaller companies can thrive on less revenue because they have less overhead. Yes, the doors are opening for small companies to enter into this space to compete with the big boys; not only in the university world at large, but also within physical therapy.

There is another door opening as well, and behind it is an opportunity for individuals with specialized knowledge to share their skills and experience directly with a community of followers with no textbook company, large or small, in the middle. And it's all happening online.

What does it take to be a physical therapy educator? This isn't the right question to ask, but we'll answer it: all physical therapist are educators. We teach patients functional skills and exercises everyday. A better question to ask is this: what does it take to be a physical therapist educator that develops a following among physical therapists?

To get an answer, we'll look at the professional journey of two therapists who are both world-renowned educators, though not at the university setting. Lenny Macrina and Mike Reinold share a similar path, and even today they work together. Their contributions to the field can be measured in pages and pages of professional journal articles and hours of online materials and webinars.

There are lots of educators in the PT world, but Lenny and Mike are unique because of how they are utilizing the Internet to teach, and how it is working to provide income.

First, let's look at the path that Lenny took to get to now.

Lenny Macrina, MSPT, SCS, CSCS, earned his physical therapy degree from Boston University. He worked with Kevin Wilk at the American Sports Medicine Institute, in Birmingham, Alabama. He has worked with professional athletes and assisted with spring training for the Tampa Bay Rays baseball organization for ten years. He has published articles in many professional journals, including *AJSM, JOSPT, Journal of Sports Health, Journal of Athletic Training, CORR, Operative Techniques in Sports Medicine,* and many others. Lenny has been presenting continuing education courses all around the United States since 2006.

Lenny has eight different continuing education courses that are available through a popular online subscription-based provider of continuing education for physical and occupational therapists as well as athletic trainers.

Now, let's look at Mike's story.

Mike Reinold, PT, DPT, SCS, ATC, CSCS began his career with a bachelor's degree in physical therapy from Northeastern University and a doctorate from Massachusetts General Hospital Institute of Health Professions, both in Boston. He pursued fellowship training, and graduated from the post-professional sports physical therapy fellowship program of the American Sports Medicine Institute, in Birmingham, Alabama, under the direction of Kevin Wilk, PT, DPT, and James Andrews, MD.

In time, Mike became the Facility Director of Champion Sports Medicine and the Coordinator of Rehabilitative Research & Clinical Education at the American Sports Medicine Institute. In addition to treating thousands of athletes from all sports and levels of play, Mike helped develop many rehabilitation protocols and return-to-sport programs that are used around the world.

Mike then left Birmingham to become the Head Athletic Trainer and Physical Therapist for the Boston Red Sox. He was part of the team when they won the World Series in 2007. He was able to influence Major League Baseball's medical model, developing a comprehensive program to address muscle imbalance and poor movement patterns before injuries develop.

Along the journey, Mike has published over fifty professional articles in journals such as *AJSM* and *JOSPT*. He is a sought-after speaker and has a long list of previous engagements.

Mike now is co-founder of Champion Physical Therapy and Performance in Waltham, Massachusetts, just outside of Boston. Still involved in baseball, he is currently a consultant to the Chicago Cubs baseball club.

In addition to all of this, the reason why we are considering Mike in this book is because of his website, www.MikeReinold.com. There, he shares his new research and clinical experience in articles read by thousands daily. His posts are translated into languages such as Spanish, Japanese, and Hungarian. He has several education products available for purchase, and a paid membership site called the "Inner Circle" where members are able to ask questions and interact with him professionally.

Several paragraphs back we asked the question: What does it take to be a physical therapist educator that develops a following among physical therapists? To be a physical therapist is to be an educator, although most of us are educators of our patients. To be *an educator of physical therapists* requires focused efforts to belong in an educational role, either as a university professor or as a continuing education provider. This will involve years of deep study and making contributions to the field. To be *an educator of physical therapists that develops a following among physical therapists* requires a life commitment to expanding the body of knowledge of physical therapy, taking the application of this knowledge base from the clinic to the world at large, and improving upon the world perception of physical therapy as a profession. Do you have to exemplify these qualities the way Mike and Lenny do? No, but it doesn't hurt.

Now that we've introduced physical therapy education as a business industry and we've introduced a couple of therapists who have involvement both in daily care and education, let's talk about how this can be a means of raising income ceilings.

Live Speaker Continuing Education

Continuing education speakers are paid to give lectures and presentations. Keynote speakers are often paid thousands of dollars to give a 90-minute talk. Best selling authors, Internet personalities, and uber-successful business leaders fetch the highest amounts—sometimes $25,000 plus— because their star power helps bring attendees to the conference. This may sound incredible, but even at this level one thing still remains true: in live presentations, the speakers are trading time for money. $25,000 for 90 minutes sounds wonderful, but there is a limit to how many talks can be given. Even at this incredible rate there is a ceiling, albeit a high one, a very high one.

Don't get too excited. Physical therapists aren't paid this much to give talks. Not at physical therapy conferences, anyway.

Let's look at the business scores of just being a live presenter/speaker at continuing education events.

Live Speaker "Raise the Ceiling" Scores

Required Overhead — This depends on how you look at it. If you only consider the technical equipment and time involvement, overhead appears very low. If you consider the additional training hours to qualify as a speaker and the cost of that training as overhead, then it could be quite high. Also consider that there is a fair amount of preparation required to give a talk or present at a conference. You can spread out the time and energy costs and reap the benefits of your efforts more if you can give the presentation more than once.

Financial Risks — Favorable. While you may count your time preparing for a presentation as overhead, you may not consider it a financial risk.

Revenue Opportunity — Neutral to Favorable.

Slowlane vs. Fastlane — Slowlane. Live talks trade time for money. This is true, even if you *love* the paycheck!

"Time for Money" vs. Passive Income — Unfavorable. If you aren't giving a talk, you aren't making money. What's more, there's just one of you, and there are only so many opportunities to present.

Scale — Neutral. Yes, you can teach a large audience at once, but you may never be able to teach that audience the same message again. Depending on how specialized your message is, there may not be that many therapists in a region that are interested enough to pay to hear it.

Time Frame To Success — Neutral. It's likely that you will be asked to give a presentation two to three months in advance. The paycheck might not come until after the event.

Long-Term Potential for Increased Income — Neutral. Teaching at conferences and providing continuing education can have a good hourly rate of pay, but there aren't opportunities to speak to audiences every day.

Potential for Sale at Exit — Unfavorable. In today's world, information that is five years old is outdated. Unless your educational products are evergreen, then the potential for someone to want to buy their rights is not exceptionally high.

	"Live Speaker" Education
Required Overhead	Neutral
Financial Risks	Favorable
Revenue Opportunity	Neutral
Slowlane vs. Fastlane	Slowlane
"Time for Money" vs. Passive Income	Neutral
Scale	Neutral
Time Frame to Success	Neutral
Longterm Potential for Increased Income	Neutral
Potential for Sale at Exit	Unfavorable

Online Continuing Education Provider

Now, let's take the concept of providing education and mix in the power of the Internet. Instead of having an event where therapists come to you, recorded material is available online and can be viewed anytime. Instead of being able to reach therapists in a single community or region for a single event, therapists all over the country and around the world can view the same education material and stream it anytime they want, day after day.

Two models exist for online continuing education. The first is for a single therapist to provide continuing education through his or her own website. In this model, all the revenue belongs to the therapist, but gaining exposure for the material is also the job of the therapist. Marketing to the masses isn't simple. If you have a household name within the profession it can be easier, but therapists looking for continuing education may not think to Google your name when they look for courses.

The second model we'll call the content hosting provider model. In it, multiple presenters and instructors provide their materials to the content hosting provider, who then offers subscriptions to the content. Medbridge is this type of business, and it is where Lenny Macrina is an instructor. Instructors only have to provide the content, and the business manages subscriptions and marketing. Instructors are paid a royalty for their materials, either a flat rate or per view. The best news for the instructor: no additional work is required, which means this can truly be passive income.

Q&A with Lenny Macrina, DPT

Lenny was kind enough to answer a few questions for this book. Here is our Q&A:

Question: You have "About" pages on two different websites, and they tell the story of how you are very active in authoring papers as well as providing physical therapy to professional teams and working alongside elite orthopedic surgeons. This is quite impressive to have only been a therapist for a little over ten years. Did all of these opportunities happen by chance, or did you actively seek them?

Answer: "As I tell most students and even other PTs, I put myself in a position to get the most out of experiences by moving to Birmingham, Alabama and associating myself with Mike Reinold and Kevin Wilk, along with Dr. Andrews, Dr. Dugas and Dr. Cain. All of these guys and many others gave me the experiences and knowledge that has helped guide me today. I am so grateful for the opportunities but knew that I could eventually control my own destiny by making connections in the industry and meeting as many people as possible."

Question: You have also been a teacher and speaker at conferences, and you have many courses available on MedBridge's online continuing education site. How does a therapist develop themselves into a presenter either for a live or online seminars?

Answer: "Again, my experiences in Birmingham allowed me to speak at local meetings, travel with Kevin Wilk to help teach at his conferences, and present at national meetings like ASMI's Injuries in Baseball or the APTA's CSM. Through this exposure and experiences, I became more comfortable and people recognized that I could help educate their staff by inviting me to speak. It has been a crazy experience, and I continually try to improve upon my courses by keeping up with the research and ways to present it in a clear and concise manner (with a little entertainment mixed in, too)."

Question: Certainly there are advantages for therapists viewing and earning continuing education units online. What has been your experience of being a presenter of online seminars? Are there advantages to being online for presenters too?

Answer: "I think some courses can be best presented in an online fashion but I always thought the experiences and lab practice time is critical. I have spoken to Medbridge about this and we are designing courses that have the viewers practice the lab portion on a friend or co-worker and have to report back to the course before they can continue on with the lecture portion. I love that clinicians can watch during their own free time, whether they're driving, riding on a train, or sitting at a pool during a weekend. It gives people access whenever they want...that's the key!"

Question: Will you compare and contrast being a speaker on MedBridge to having your own website for your content?

Answer: "As of now, Medbridge is my only mode of getting a course out to the masses. Mike Reinold and myself are in the process of putting a course out in mid 2016. We're very excited to get the content out. I do not have my own website but utilize social media: Twitter, Facebook, Instagram, our company website www.champ.pt, to push content out as blog posts or research study links. I hope people can gain a little insight into what I think may help them become a better clinician through my experiences."

Full interview with Lenny Macrina is available here.

http://bit.ly/1rvklib

Online Continuing Education Provider "Raise the Ceiling" Scores

Required Overhead — This depends. Running your own website isn't free. Getting traffic requires marketing. Blog posts don't write themselves. Promotional videos don't produce themselves. On top of that is the work to create the content for the courses. Working with an online provider of continuing education like Medbridge can have less expenses and much less ongoing involvement.

Financial Risks — Favorable. While you may count your time preparing for a presentation as overhead, you may not consider it a financial risk.

Revenue Opportunity — Neutral to Favorable. If you own the entire website and you have a lot of traffic and can convert a lot of that traffic into sales, then your revenue opportunity can be very high. Getting the same exposure as a company like Medbridge can be difficult.

Slowlane vs. Fastlane — Fastlane. Remember, Fastlane is the combination of a scalable business that doesn't trade time for money. Having your own website just for continuing education courses you teach is Fastlane, but if you can bring other instructors under your umbrella, you immediately start to scale up. In other words, providing your content yourself or through a company like Medbridge is good; growing into a company like Medbridge would be even better.

"Time for Money" vs. Passive Income — Highly Favorable. Providing knowledge through an online medium is passive income.

Scale - Highly Favorable.

Time Frame To Success — Neutral. It is true that once materials are available for purchase that money can be made immediately, but the time needed to develop the material and even to develop yourself as an instructor can be extensive.

Long-Term Potential for Increased Income — Favorable. Once your course is online, it will be there until someone takes it down. Unless your content is proven to have errors in it or unless you end your relationship with the content hosting company, this can be a long time. And for every year that passes, you'll stay young and energetic in the eyes of everyone who learns from you!

Potential for Sale at Exit — Neutral to Favorable. If you are marketing your own material, it may only have a shelf life of 3-5 years. This will be less desirable to own if you are not part of the business, adding new material. If the business has many contributors and systems to add new courses, and if there are strong numbers of subscribers that create a recurring revenue stream, then acquisition desirability will be much higher.

	Online Continuing Education Provider
Required Overhead	Neutral
Financial Risks	Favorable
Revenue Opportunity	Favorable
Slowlane vs. Fastlane	Fastlane
"Time for Money" vs. Passive Income	Highly Favorable
Scale	Highly Favorable
Time Frame to Success	Neutral
Longterm Potential for Increased Income	Favorable
Potential for Sale at Exit	Favorable

Online Platform for Continuing Education

Continuing education courses are not the only way knowledge is shared. Professional journals and peer-reviewed articles are a staple of the physical therapy body of knowledge. These can be viewed online, of course, sometimes with a society membership. Authors and researchers can also make their content available through blogs and email lists, which creates a unique business opportunity that we will discuss now.

The Internet provides many opportunities, but convincing buyers to purchase is not simple. The first thing that has to happen is the message has to get to them. There are several prominent Internet sales and marketing experts who focus their entire business on teaching how to maximize Internet sales. Perry Marshall, Michael Hyatt, Jeff Walker, and Russell Brunson are a few of the major players. Here are a few of the points they teach:

- Having an email list is a license to print money. —Jeff Walker

- 20% of your customers will bring 80% of your revenue. — Perry Marshall

- To build an online business, you need a platform. — Michael Hyatt

- A sales "funnel" is the key to high profits. — Russell Brunson

Just for a moment, let's depart from the world of PT to dive into these concepts and illustrate their power.

The Pareto Principle, which was published in 1896, states that for many events 80% of the effects come from 20% of the causes. Pareto observed that 80% of the land in Italy was owned by 20% of the population, and that 20% of the peapods in his garden contained 80% of the peas. The same holds true for us today. For example, 80% of the population drives on 20% of the roads, and 20% of items in grocery stores are routinely purchased by 80% of shoppers.

This rough mathematical formula is called a power law. Perry Marshall describes in his book, *80/20 Sales and Marketing,* that if we are given an average number and a sample size, we can use this power law to determine extremes. For instance, if 50,000 people spend $100 for a football ticket, we can calculate how many will spend over $10,000 for something high-end, like a skybox. The formula also shows that for every one million people who spend $5.00 at Starbucks, a few people will spend $2,000.00(!), not necessarily on coffee, but on a high-end espresso machine.

The Pareto Principle can be applied to everything in life. 80% of our results come from 20% of our efforts. The hard part is figuring out which 20% gets us the results we need. Once we have this isolated, pouring 100% of our effort into the right thing will yield exponentially higher results.

When it comes to the Internet, there are many trailblazers who have spent years finding the 20% of methods that work the best. The number one recommendation at present is to build an email list of people who are interested in your products or services. To do this, you need to build a platform where they can find you.

What is a platform? It starts with a niche. The Internet is full of generalized products competing for our interest. We are so overwhelmed with "general" that we hardly pay attention to it. For example, a website promoting children's stories might not interest many people, but a website promoting stories with characters who are girls adopted from China has a good chance of finding a niche audience that will return to that website again and again.

A platform will have: a website where people can find you, a blog where you provide free content to grow and interact with your audience, possibly connections to social media, and, most importantly, a method of collecting email addresses. A "monetized" platform will have products or services that are for sale.

I just described something as general an automobile, but you know there are trucks and cars and motorcycles. You know there are Ferraris and Toyotas. And under the hood of each are thousands of components, all that can have different forms to serve different purposes. What works best? What are the 20% that provide the best results? Michael Hyatt is the expert at this. His book *Platform* is the place to start learning about this.

Why is a platform so important? Because, according to Jeff Walker, "having an email list is having a license to print money."

What is it about an email list that makes it so great? An email list should be a group of people who already have interests in what your platform promotes. You don't have to focus on *finding* customers when you have an email list; you can focus on *selling to them*.

Getting a customer to buy a product involves a lot of psychology. There are impulse decisions for things that cost a few dollars. Things that cost hundreds of dollars are bought on impulse too, but a lot more work goes into priming the customer to make that decision. Jeff Walker's book *Launch* describes how we can pique our customers' interest, build their confidence in us and our company, and get them to not only buy from us, but also to promote us to their friends. He does this with a series of messages and videos that he sends out to his email list, each message having a specific purpose to teach and build trust, and eventually, sell. It works. His techniques have been used in multi-million dollar product launches. Now, he launches his own training program, where he teaches people who sell their wares online how to use his techniques. Essentially, he has condensed the top techniques for selling—his 20%—into a repeatable method.

Don't have a list? No problem. Rent another person's list. Products are often launched with what is called a joint venture, or an affiliate launch, where the person who has a list will promote a product, then receive some of the profits from purchases that came from people on their list.

As strange as it may sound, the best time to sell to a person is right after they have bought from you. At that point in time, their defenses are down and they believe in what they just bought. Russell Brunson describes "sales funnels" that are proven methods for making an additional offer to a person who just purchased. For instance, if a person just purchased a three-month supply of a vitamin supplement, they are very likely to buy a six-month's supply right then if a 25% discount is given. The timing of this offer generates a tremendous amount of sales. This is another example of a small tweak, far less than 20% of our effort, that produces tremendous results.

How does all of this tie into physical therapy and raising income ceilings? It shows that there is a lot of power generating income online. A lot of this can be passive income as well. Don't be deceived—it's not as easy. Setting up a website and walking away won't work. It takes effort. Jeff Walker, Perry Marshall, and Michael Hyatt all post new content on their blogs daily. Daily. But they also have income well above typical physical therapist salaries.

There is strong potential for therapists to build a platform and realize additional income through the Internet, too.

Earlier, we introduced Mike Reinold. Mike's website, www.MikeReinold.com, has a blog where he posts new content on regular basis. He has recently launched a podcast as well. Both have content he has written, but they also include content from other therapists. Mike provides high-quality, clinical information, often with research article abstracts and strength and conditioning tips that are easy to apply.

Unique to Mike's website is a subscription membership. Members get access to even more content, live webinars, and interaction with Mike. This is available at a very affordable price point.

From a business standpoint, this subscription website gives Mike recurring passive income. He only has one level of membership, but with his audience spreading across multiple countries there is potential for large numbers of members. Many Internet teachers offer "master level" memberships for higher premiums, or offer courses or webinars at higher prices. Remember, there are people who are able and willing to spend $10,000 to see a football game, or $2,000 at Starbucks. Mike isn't doing this today, but his platform provides the opportunity.

Q&A with Mike Reinold, DPT

I had a chance to ask Mike a few questions about his business. Here's what he had to say:

Question: From the information on your "About" page on your website, www.MikeReinold.com, it's clear that early on you began developing your knowledge and specialization within PT. Will you describe the moment when you decided to take your knowledge and make it available online?

Answer: "I started my path towards education early in my career by traveling to speak at national conferences and teaching weekend seminars. When I took a job in Major League Baseball, it was very consuming and took away my ability to travel to teach. I decided that I can provide the same, if not better, educational opportunities online in the form of my website. I essentially decided to start a site to share what I am currently learning myself with others."

Question: Did the idea for Inner Circle come first, or did that come after you started building your platform?

Answer: "My Inner Circle came over time as my audience was looking for more information to consume. I thought having a smaller group of people that were really into learning from me would be a great opportunity, and it really has turned out to be fun."

Question: You're a speaker at conferences, your website and blog have won awards for their quality, and you've just launched a podcast. You're very driven, and your platform is already positioned to give you great reach into the physical therapy community. What are your goals for the Inner Circle?

Answer: "My goals for my Inner Circle, and all my other products and offerings, is simple. I want to educate and share what I am currently learning with others. When this is sincerely your objective, the business aspect of the website works out."

Full interview with Mike Reinold is available here.

http://bit.ly/1XxeTsP

Online Platform for Clinical Education "Raise the Ceiling" Scores

Required Overhead — Just as with the previous section, it depends. Running a website isn't free. Getting traffic requires marketing. Blog posts don't write themselves. Promotional videos don't produce themselves. On top of that is the work to create the content for the courses.

Financial Risk — Favorable. The out-of-pocket expense to run a website is relatively low, but the time and skill needed to run one can be high. It is possible to gradually increase the complexity of your website over time and keep the overall costs low.

Revenue Opportunity — Favorable to Highly Favorable. Internet sales coaches say that having an email list is "a license to print money."

Slowlane vs. Fastlane — Fastlane. 100% Fastlane.

"Time for Money" vs. Passive Income — Highly Favorable. Providing knowledge through an online medium is passive income. That's not to say that it doesn't require time. I'm sure Mike would tell you that it takes a LOT of time. However, blog posts and podcasts can be batch produced. With practice, a month's worth of content can be generated in only a few hours.

Time Frame To Success — Neutral. The variables here are having a list and knowing how to get sales conversions. How quickly can you build a list? Is it possible to buy lists from other people? Once you have the list, do you have content and unique sales propositions in place that convert traffic into revenue? This is not what we are taught in PT school, but we all have different experiences in life. The experiences you bring to the table can determine how quickly you can have success.

Long-Term Potential for Increased Income — Favorable. Not every blog makes money. Those that provide value to the most people at a favorable price point can have great success. That being said, even Internet leaders like Michael Hyatt and Jeff Walker describe their success coming after years of effort. Much time will be needed for platforms to be established and online business skills honed. Growth can be linear for a period, then it can explode exponentially.

Potential for Sale at Exit — Neutral. The hope of all Internet platform builders is to establish passive income that will last well into life's golden years. Could a website business be acquired and rebranded in the future by a new company? Absolutely. The trouble is that in our day and time information is outdated once it's a few months old. What systems will be in place within the business to ensure the release of new material after the owner/founder is gone? These will influence acquisition.

	Online Platform for Clinical Education
Required Overhead	Neutral
Financial Risks	Favorable
Revenue Opportunity	Favorable
Slowlane vs. Fastlane	Fastlane
"Time for Money" vs. Passive Income	Highly Favorable
Scale	Highly Favorable
Time Frame to Success	Neutral
Longterm Potential for Increased Income	Favorable
Potential for Sale at Exit	Neutral

Self-Publishing

Another form of providing education is writing books. With consistent effort and know-how, authors can create book platforms that reach patient and therapist readers all around the world, generating passive income.

By many accounts, traditional book publishing is dead, but new mechanisms exist for individuals to self-publish. During a podcast interview between Entrepreneur on Fire host John Lee Dumas and Shark Tank superstar Barbara Corcoran, Barbara said that she only made about fifty cents per sale of her book, *Shark Tales*. John Lee Dumas told her about how Tim Ferriss's book, *The 4-Hour Chef*, was selling on Amazon and that Tim was getting seven dollars per book. Barbara was stunned! When a shark's jaw drops, you know it's good intel!

The Internet and digital books make this possible. Just as with continuing education, an author can sell to an audience that finds his or her website, or through an online marketplace like the Amazon Kindle Store, the Apple iBookstore, or Barnes & Noble. Professional cover designers, editors, and formatters can be hired from all over the world for low costs. In some cases having a printed book is necessary, and several print-on-demand services are available that will print a book for a small fee.

It's possible to learn about self-publishing from several sources. There are books written about self-publishing in general, and books that focus on specific platforms like Amazon Kindle. Many podcasts are available for "Indie" (independent) authors that give outstanding ideas for turning self-published books into a profitable business. There is also Self-Publishing School (which I joined while writing this book) that teaches and guides students from start to finish through the writing process, providing coaches and a supportive online community of writers.

Q&A with Sean Sumner, DPT

Sean Sumner is a Senior Physical Therapist at UC Davis Medical Center in Sacramento, California. He is the best-selling of two Amazon Kindle books, *Sciatica: Low Back Pain Relief Once And For All*, and *Neck Check: Chronic Neck Pain Relief Once and For Al*l. Sean is also the Online Community Manager for Self-Publishing School. Sean spoke with me and answered a few questions for this book. Here is our Q&A about self-publishing.

Question: How did you get started writing books? Where did you get the vision?

Answer: "I got started writing books mainly because I wanted to create a revenue stream from passive income. I don't have this really big altruistic vision of wanting to help people, even though that's a good part of my books. The real reason I started writing is I want to create some passive income. My goal has always been for my wife to be able to cut down to part-time or less, and be with the kids a little more often. Right now we're both working full-time. So, my entire goal is to find a way that I can get some passive income coming in but I don't have to devote more hours away from the family, but I can still have that revenue coming in.

I looked around at all kinds of different ways to do that. Initially I started a podcast. I tried blogging. I tried lots of different things that a lot of gurus were telling me to do. And so finally I said, you know, that's not giving me immediate revenue, that may take years to build up. So, I decided to write a book. I had seen some people really doing well on Amazon. I decided to go ahead and write a book and on a subject matter that I know really well, and see how it does. And that's what I did. Ever since then, that's been the direction I've been heading—to write more books as a way of getting more passive income. It's been really successful for me so far, and I'm hoping to continue with it."

Question: You have two books available on Amazon, and both are on spinal issues. How did you arrive at these topics?

Answer: "The topics I chose for my books is because that's what I know. I give the same speech to patients when they come in on their first visit. We discuss their anatomy and I go over all of the basic things. I've had so many people say, " Man, if I had just known that three weeks ago that would have really helped out. You did a really good job of explaining it." People tell me that they looked online to find information but they didn't know what to trust and what not to trust. I decided to take that basic information and put it out in a book and see how people respond to it. That's how I started. I started writing what I felt confident in.

My fear was that another physical therapist would tell me, "That's a load of crap…why are you telling people that?" The response I got from therapists was, "Wow, that's great! I'm so happy for you." That fear I had which limited me for a while, none of that ever really came through."

Question: You earned the OCS certification and have experience lecturing to physicians and physical therapists, but your books are written to consumers, not healthcare providers. Do you think your special training and teaching experience was necessary to write your books?

Answer: "I don't think so. Does it help me gain a little bit of an edge over someone who might not have those qualifications in their author page? Maybe. It does help establish my credibility, and that lets readers read the book with more confidence. But do I think having certifications are necessary to be a author? Absolutely not. I work with people all the time who write books who don't have a high level of authority in their field and they do well with their books. For physical therapists specifically, I think just having a physical therapy degree and having clinical experience is enough."

Question: Within the self-publishing world, there are beginners who might make a few hundred dollars with a book, then there are "authorpreneurs" who make $30,000 a month with e-books. How much of an opportunity do you think exists for therapists?

Answer: "I think you have the whole range. I'm working with a gentleman right now who is probably going to make a couple hundred dollars a month on his book. He knows that going into it. His strategy isn't to make money, it's to become an authority for his audience, which is home health therapists. When he goes to do a talk to a home health physical therapy company he'll have a best selling book on Amazon on the subject.

There's another gentleman, a physical therapist, who is planning to make a few thousands dollars, but the book is to serve a back end program that is already selling $30,000 a month. Books can do many things. What you make depends on how you position them. If you're just going strictly on book sales, what you will make depends on how many books you plan on writing and how much appeal the subject matter has.

I think it's reasonable, if you have a few books out, to be making anywhere from $1,000 to $4,000 a month. That is, if you have four to five books out and you do well with a particular subject. If you just put one book out and you don't have a great subject or a great audience then it will be hard to make those numbers. It's just like any other business industry. If you have one book and it's well received, then you've built an audience who would probably buy another book from you. It takes work, though, just like any other avenue. Some of those avenues, you've got to put the hours in. With this one, I put the hours in and wrote the book and it just continually sells. Even if I don't do anything I'm going to get a check from Amazon because the book continues to sell. That's the great benefit of passive income."

Question: Are there places where therapists can go to learn about self-publishing?

Answer: There are a lot of places with information, but only a few that are really where you should be looking. I can tell you from experience. I tried several packages, and I didn't get my book out. The best one out there is the one I associate myself with, and that is Self-Publishing School by Chandler Bolt. I've received the best education from it, as well as great contacts and connections. It was a step-by-step process that guided me through how to do it.

I put out a book before going through SPS and it did okay. Then I went though Chandler's program and learned how to do it the right way, with a professional cover and professional editing and better marketing. Now, my book has done much better. It's an education. With any of my other books, I'll go right back through the same process."

Full interview with Sean Sumner is available here

http://bit.ly/28Oc22S

Self-Publishing "Raise the Ceiling" Scores

Required Overhead — Neutral to Favorable. Books require time to write. There is expense in self-publishing school, but it's comparable to many PT continuing education courses. Professional editing and cover design can cost a few hundred dollars per book.

Financial Risk — Favorable. The out of pocket expense to self-publish a book is relatively low.

Revenue Opportunity — Neutral to Highly Favorable. One book that is not well received might not generate much revenue. A book series that gains popularity can be very profitable.

Slowlane vs. Fastlane — Fastlane.

"Time for Money" vs. Passive Income — Highly Favorable. Revenue that comes from self-publishing is passive income. Yes, time is involved in writing books, but once they are published, little work is required.

Time Frame To Success — Favorable to Highly Favorable. The variables here are writing a good book and getting some professional help in just the right stages of the self-publishing process. How quickly can you write a series? Some independent authors publish five to ten books per year, all while working a full-time job. The effort you put into self-publishing, the quality of that effort, and the results of your marketing will determine your time frame to success.

Longterm Potential for Increased Income — Favorable. Not every book makes money. A series of books is more likely to succeed than a single volume. Authors that provide strong value to many people over a long period of time can have great success. Audiences will have to be built, which takes time and effort. Growth can be linear for a period, then it can explode exponentially.

Potential for Sale at Exit — Neutral. We are at the dawn of the digital publishing era. It is hard to know what will become of book businesses in years to come. As technologies change, books with stories and anecdotes rooted in current times and technology will become outdated and antiquated, and will see their sales evaporate. Books that focus on evergreen principles are more likely to stand the test of time, as long as they aren't rooted out by the latest best sellers. Books can be lead magnets for larger businesses, which have more potential for sale at exit.

	Self-Publishing
Required Overhead	Neutral
Financial Risks	Favorable
Revenue Opportunity	Favorable
Slowlane vs. Fastlane	Fastlane
"Time for Money" vs. Passive Income	Highly Favorable
Scale	Highly Favorable
Time Frame to Success	Favorable
Longterm Potential for Increased Income	Favorable
Potential for Sale at Exit	Neutral

Physical Therapy Business Consulting

Another area of education that therapists can provide online involves business skills, particularly those relating to niche markets like solo practices, cash-based practices, and independent home health practices. Certainly, this information lends itself to blogs, podcasts, and email lists. Providing excellent content and building a platform with quality posts and podcasts will establish an audience and attract newcomers who are interested in the subject matter. In order to turn this into income, a product or service has to be sold. Online business education experts sell books and consulting services through their websites.

First, let's look at consulting as a profession. How does a therapist establish themselves as a consultant? Does it take a significant amount of experience? Yes, but you can't put a number of years on it. What is more important is having a deep understanding of how the therapy business works for a given area of practice, as well as having the ability to quickly grasp the big picture of organizations and spot problem areas that need attention. Does this sound familiar? It is exactly what therapists do for patients during initial evaluations. The difference, of course, is that the business is the patient. Consultants who are worth their expensive rates are able to identify a few key changes that, if fully executed, will increase business performance. To go back to the Pareto Principle, consultants look for the 20% that will affect the 80% in the most positive way.

Establishing credibility is critical for consultants. A strong client list may be the best way to do this. Getting started can be more difficult. In today's world this can hardly be done without a website. Existing clients and new customers will want to see a steady stream of value-added content coming from a consultant. Speaking at conferences is also a method for getting exposure.

Consultants are paid either by a flat fee for a site visit, or by the hour. After a visit, they can be kept on retainer for a monthly fee. With this ongoing relationship, practices can have access to the consultant for accountability, sending monthly reports for review, and can ask questions as they work through the changes given during their site visit. Depending on the desires of the business, consultants can do site visits every one to two years. Oversight and assistance can range from business analytics to documentation audits to regulatory compliance.

While you might think that being a consultant is still a "time for money" exchange, the services offered by consultants within healthcare are very scalable. Books, webinars, software, and subscription services are options for business development that will create passive income.

Physical Therapy Business Consulting "Raise the Ceiling" Scores

Required Overhead — There's a common trend here: it depends. Running a high-powered website isn't free. Blog posts don't magically appear. Traffic doesn't happen by itself. Have a great idea for some software? A business owner friend of mine has over $700,000 tied up in software development.

Financial Risks — Neutral. How much you spend on development determines your risks.

Revenue Opportunity — Favorable to Highly Favorable. Consultants should charge high rates. What is valued more: a Corolla or a Land Cruiser? If you think you'll get more business by lowering your rates, you might. But you will also have to deal with cheap business owners. Higher rates equal higher margins. Earn the right to stay on retainer and return for another site visit in one to two years. This can snowball into a strong revenue stream that has a large passive component to it. On top of this, many educational products are scalable.

Slowlane vs. Fastlane — Mostly Fastlane.

"Time for Money" vs. Passive Income — Neutral to Favorable. Providing business-consulting services on site is trading time for money. However, many products that complement a consulting business are purely passive in nature.

Time Frame To Success — Neutral. Like PRN work, getting a consulting gig brings in income immediately. Building a sustainable business with large passive income components will take much, much longer.

Long-Term Potential for Increased Income — Favorable. Building a client list builds momentum.

Potential for Sale at Exit: Neutral. Recurring value of the business will determine potential for sale. Some medical consulting firms generate tremendous revenue and have multiple locations across the country. If the business consists of a solo consultant that trades time for money, then potential for acquisition could be low.

	PT Business Consulting
Required Overhead	Neutral
Financial Risks	Neutral
Revenue Opportunity	Favorable
Slowlane vs. Fastlane	Fastlane
"Time for Money" vs. Passive Income	Neutral
Scale	Highly Favorable
Time Frame to Success	Neutral
Longterm Potential for Increased Income	Favorable
Potential for Sale at Exit	Neutral

Physical Therapy Business Education

Now let's look at Physical Therapy Business Education. That is essentially what this book is about, not nuts and bolts within a niche, but a high-level view of many different business models. Therapists need business education because, frankly, it isn't and shouldn't be the focus of physical therapy school. There is simply too much clinical information that needs to be mastered to dive into business at a deep level during school. With each area of practice having unique opportunities and challenges, and with these changing year after year, it would take a lot of time away from clinical education for this material to be in PT programs.

This void in business training coupled with the income ceiling within therapy creates opportunity for those with expertise to teach business techniques. Therapists who have their own businesses or who are thinking about business want information. The more niche based, the better chance an educational product has at having a long shelf life.

Creating a website, writing blog posts, developing an email list, hosting a podcast—all of these platform-building steps are part of the educating process, but this type of content is generally given away for free. Business education can be delivered in book form, or through a number of different Internet media methods.

Providing business education without consulting services can lend itself to one-time purchases. This being the case, a book or a course could be a one-time sale. Charge too little and you won't see much return on your investment of time spent writing the book. You'll also send a signal that the book is not very valuable. Charge too much and you might not sell very many books. Keep this in mind, though: therapists are accustomed to paying a few hundred dollars for a continuing education course. A book with lots of details about how to run a niche business can have a much higher price tag than a work of fiction.

Even for physical therapy business education, digital publishing can be the best option. First, the financial barrier to entry is very low. The marketplace for people looking for digital books is growing. Profits from digital books are strong, with Amazon Kindle paying a good royalty. The advantage of an online digital bookstore is that readers go there to buy, as long as these pricing tiers are attractive to you. It is possible to sell your book on your own website, but you will forfeit a lot of traffic. If your book is very niche-based, word of mouth and therapist referrals can generate sales. Furthermore, if you want to charge a higher amount (recommended if you provide a lot of detail), then you will want to keep all of the revenue from the book, not share a percentage with Amazon.

It is worth noting that the size of the market will determine how many books you can sell. There are high numbers of physical therapists in the world, but only a few of these will be interested in niche-based business skills.

Are there ways to get more traction out of a single book/course?

Yes.

In the early 2000's, Bill Phillips wrote a book called *Body for Life*. It was one of the first times when eating six small meals a day as opposed to three large meals was introduced. In the book, Phillips recommended using dietary supplements like protein shakes and vitamins and supplements that his company, EAS Sports Nutrition, sold. The book sold 3.5 million copies. This type of volume can net an author millions, but Phillips eventually sold his supplement company for more than $100 million.

Books and courses are business in and of themselves, but both can also be on-ramps to other business products or services. Developing the "back-end" of a book business is a way to capitalize on the momentum of a book. Speaking engagements, coaching, live events, membership sites, and product sales are ways to add revenue.

Jarod Carter, DPT, whom we met with earlier in the book and is the author of the niche-based business book *Medicare & Cash-Pay Physical Therapy*, answered this question in our interview that relates to this topic:

Question: For physical therapists, running a cash-based practice is outside of the box, but having an online business is taking entrepreneurialism to another level. What inspired you to go down this road, to write your ebook, start your blog and your websites?

Answer: "I've just always had the entrepreneurial bug. I've always felt driven in that direction. On top of that, since I got into the workforce, I've never felt that one single source of income was a safe bet.

Even if you're in the healthcare realm, where there's always going to be a lot of work for all of us, you never know what's going to happen to your health or your body. There are so many different things that could happen that if you only rely on one single string of income, you could really get hammered.

So, those two reasons together: wanting to be entrepreneurial and then having more than one stream of income. A third reason would be that I wanted income streams that were not reliant on my physical presence. That they're truly passive or at least that they would be mobile, virtual, so I could run my Internet-based business from anywhere in the world. Those were the three driving factors that pushed me into seeking out side businesses."

Full interview with Jarod Carter is available here
http://bit.ly/1UpUPFl

Aaron LeBauer, DPT, also has a PT business ebook and a consulting service. He answered a question on this topic during our interview:

Question: In addition to providing physical therapy services, you also work as a consultant to other therapy practices, and your Cash PT Toolkit is available for sale online. No doubt, you have targets that you hope to achieve. What are your goals for your business(es) and, more importantly, will you describe where you were when you came to have these goals?

Answer: "My goal—because I can only help so many people in a day— is to help other physical therapists to help more patients, so that way *I* can help more patients. It's a way to kind of multiply myself and help other people help more patients. Rather than seeing five people an hour, I can help other PTs start practices that provide quality care and I feel like I'm doing something useful.

You know, the other goal in there is that, you know, it's fun. Instead of telling the same thing, saying over and over again how I do this or that, I put it in a blog. I created a course, and a couple of things to download, like the toolkit. It does create an alternative stream of income. But at the same time, it's more about helping more people achieve the same thing I did. There was no one there helping people when I started and the information wasn't readily available."

Full interview with Aaron LeBauer is available here
http://bit.ly/1ZZKsK6

Physical Therapy Business Education "Raise the Ceiling" Scores

Required Overhead — Neutral. There are self-publishing methods available that are very low cost. The same can be said for hosting an online course. Writing a book, creating a course, learning how to use the tools to accomplish the tasks takes time.

Financial Risks — Favorable. Writing a self-published ebook has very low financial risks, other than required writing time. The same can be said of an online course.

Revenue Opportunity — Neutral. Writing a book does not equate with becoming a best-selling author. One-time purchase items still create passive income, but the size of markets could limit total revenue. Live teaching in person or with webinars might present the same content and material in a course format that will bring a higher price point.

Slowlane vs. Fastlane — Fastlane, though scalability may be limited by niche sizes.

"Time for Money" vs. Passive Income — Neutral to Favorable. Creating content takes time. However, it can be done on your own schedule. I get my writing done early in the morning, before the kids wake up. Once the book is complete and is available for purchase online, the income from book sales is passive.

Scale - Highly Favorable. The World Wide Web is just that: worldwide.

Time Frame To Success — Unfavorable to Neutral. How quickly can you write a book or create a course? The first draft of this book took two months to complete. Jarod Carter said his first book took him nine months. Sales depend on how much momentum for the book you were able to generate at the time for launch. Entire workshops are designed just for this (Jeff Walker's Product Launch Formula, Self-Publishing School). Hal Elrod, bestselling author of *The Miracle Morning*, said his book did not begin to sell well until two years after his launch. He continued to promote it the entire time.

Long-Term Potential for Increased Income — Neural to Favorable. It's not the norm for one book to create sustained income year after year. Authors write more books and try to expand their audiences with each release. Some books do well; others flop. It's not easy to gain or maintain a readership that will provide recurring revenue. Focused, continual effort is required to achieve at a high level.

	PT Business Education
Required Overhead	Neutral
Financial Risks	Favorable
Revenue Opportunity	Neutral
Slowlane vs. Fastlane	Fastlane
"Time for Money" vs. Passive Income	Highly Favorable
Scale	Highly Favorable
Time Frame to Success	Unfavorable
Longterm Potential for Increased Income	Neutral
Potential for Sale at Exit	Neutral

Physical Therapy Software Services

Another area open for innovation and development within the profession of physical therapy is computer software and computer-based services. This can be a multitude of different things. It could be global software that serves as the backbone of a practice, that therapists use as their electronic medical record and billing systems. It could be more specific, and provide an excellent home exercise programs. These are two types common to PT, but within the healthcare field there are also companies that build software programs that serve as add-ons to larger EMRs, or that provide polished workflows for certain aspects of patient interaction. Here are some examples:

- Software designed specifically to email patients their bill and allow online bill payment

- Billing statement companies that add a code onto the patient's statement and allow online bill payment

- Software for automated, kiosk-style patient registration and insurance eligibility checks
- Software to record marketing efforts and track referral patterns to determine the success of those efforts

- Local and remote computer support companies for networks, hardware, and software

- Hosting companies that will place your servers in the cloud and provide backup of all data

- HIPAA training and compliance platforms that provide education and house employee handbooks and training records.

All of these options are possibilities for development within physical therapy, but the market size is considerably smaller for it than it is for all of medicine. Great care is needed to make sure the right developments are made that will interest and benefit therapists while also providing opportunities for growth and expansion for the software company.

What does it takes for a software company to make money? To get therapist's attention, a need must be met for the first time or in a unique way. To keep business, the user interface must be refined and simple enough that it is easy to use, and back end processes must run flawlessly enough that there aren't many support calls. To be profitable, pricing must not be a barrier to purchase, and all support and services must stay within budgeted parameters. For the software to expand and have growth, therapists must enjoy using it, or there must be some savings of time, energy, or money that make it a necessity.

Sound easy?

Let's look at the story of two software companies that were founded and led by physical therapists: WebPT and SimpleSet.net.

WebPT is a hosted electronic medical record and billing platform. Their "About" page provides this description:

Simpleset.net is a home exercise program web application, designed by physical therapists. They are based out of Saskatoon, Saskatchewan in Canada. Eric Gartner, one of the founders, was glad to answer some questions for this book.

185

Q&A with Eric Gartner, MPT

Question: What is the origin story of SimpleSet?

Answer: "SimpleSet was founded in 2009 by Travis Brunn, Eric Gartner, Robert Hydomako, and Neal Zaluski. Travis had the idea while spending a year away from physiotherapy. He noticed that there was a big need for technology within physiotherapy, particularly when it came to exercise prescription software. While there were a few options on the market, they didn't reflect the advanced capabilities of what well-written software could do at that time.

The four of us had been classmates in Physiotherapy school. As part of this process, we had the opportunity to work with each other on a variety of projects. We recognized our complementary skillsets and similar approaches to physiotherapy, and thought it would be a good mix for bringing an innovative solution to the market."

Question: With four PTs as founders, where did you find coding expertise?

Answer: "Travis had a previous life as a software developer. After 11 years as a professional coder, he decided to take on a new challenge and become a physical therapist. He is a one-man show in that department and does all the coding himself. He won't like me saying this, but he's brilliant."

Question: Running a software company is not something you learn how to do in PT school. What is the biggest challenge you have faced and how did you deal with it?

Answer: "As with most small businesses, our biggest challenges are marketing and customer acquisition. We are learning more and more as we go, through research, mentors, and other industry professionals. We recognize our expertise is in the clinical setting, and learning from others is important. In some ways, we can take our experiences from the clinic and apply them to our company. For example, much like clinical practice, we want to learn about our population needs, implement a well thought out strategy (marketing for instance), find a way to measure its impact, adjust based on the findings and repeat. The critical thinking skills you learn throughout university come in handy in many areas of life."

Question: The reach of the Internet allows tremendous scale. Is SimpleSet being used in interesting places? How did your message find these locations?

Answer: "We have users in countries all over the world, and one place that has surprised us is Iceland. We have a large contingent of passionate users in Iceland. Physiotherapy is usually a relatively small, tight-knit community in each country, and word of mouth in Iceland has taken us into a population we couldn't have anticipated. Pretty neat, actually."

Question: What goals do you have for your company, and more importantly, when did you come to have them?

Answer: "Our primary goal remains the same as when we started—to advance the software capability involved in the clinic-therapist-patient interaction. Our lives and our patients' lives increasingly rely on technology to simplify complex situations. We believe we have a unique perspective to improve these situations."

Full interview with Eric Gartner is available here

http://bit.ly/23jiScL

The Story of WebPT

In 2006, Heidi Jannenga, a leading sports physical therapist and clinic director, was looking for ways to improve her clinic's bottom line. After identifying dictation as well as paper documentation management as two of her practice's biggest costs, she started looking for a less expensive solution to documentation and enlisted the help of then-boyfriend Brad Jannenga, a seasoned technologist who had experience in software development. Heidi knew she needed something that would not only fit her workflow as a PT, but also would be affordable, easy to use, and a cinch to implement in her clinic. The more Brad and Heidi shopped around, though, the more discouraged they became. That was when they decided to partner and develop her clinic's dream solution. Brad started going to work with Heidi to get an idea of her workflow and documentation needs. In the evenings, the two would regroup and brainstorm on how the software should work. Then, Brad would get to coding and Heidi would get to testing. And piece by piece, WebPT—a web-based physical therapy EMR—was born.

Heidi and Brad officially launched the software in 2008 (and got married). Within three years, their cloud-based idea grew into the leading physical therapy software on the market. Today, as president and co-founder, Heidi leads WebPT's product vision, branding efforts, and company culture, while advocating for the physical therapy profession on a national scale. Since its launch, WebPT has evolved from a startup into one of the nation's fastest-growing privately held companies, providing more than 200 local jobs in Phoenix, while helping more than 50,000 members achieve greatness in therapy practice.

In addition to offering defensible, compliant, and intuitive documentation, WebPT provides physical therapists, occupational therapists, and speech-language pathologists with intelligent business reporting, interactive and organized scheduling, integrated billing, and one-stop shopping (and saving) with the WebPT Marketplace. And it's all web-based, which means therapists can document, schedule, and bill anywhere, anytime.

In spite of her busy schedule, Heidi Jannenga was kind enough to field some questions from me. Her answers are incredible.

Q&A with Heidi Jannenga, DPT

Question: We just read the origin story of WebPT that is on your "About page", but what is the behind-the-scenes story about how many hours you worked each week and how long it took to develop a viable product?

Answer: "I was the clinic director for three physical therapy clinics in Tempe, Arizona, and as part of my role, I was responsible for P&L (profit and loss). In an effort to maintain a healthy bottom line in the face of declining reimbursements, I started reviewing all of our expenses to look for opportunities where we could reduce our operational costs. At that time, our biggest expense was transcription and dictation. I knew that many of our referring physicians were transitioning to EMRs, so I asked my then-boyfriend, Brad (who also happened to be a technologist), to help me find something for my practice. When we couldn't find anything worthwhile or affordable, we decided to put our heads together and build something—something that was only supposed to be for my clinics. During that process, I continued to work full-time as a clinician and clinic director, and Brad—who had just sold some e-commerce stores he had built approximately nine months prior—began programming version one of WebPT.

During normal clinic hours, Brad shadowed me to get a feel for my workflow. On the days he didn't shadow me, he'd write code. Then we'd meet during the evenings to go over plans for the following day, and I would QA the work we'd already completed. This cycle went on and on for about nine months. As a single-income household in the heart of the recession, Brad and I definitely stuck to a pretty strict budget. We didn't go out much, we ate lots of peanut butter and jelly sandwiches, and our vacation getaways were camping trips. Once I actually started using the application at work, we gathered feedback from my staff and talked about how we could alter or enhance the product. So, it was an iterative process from the very beginning, but combined, we were spending more time creating WebPT than someone would spend at a full-time job—and all of the hours I put into creating our product fell on top of my primary job at the clinic. About 10 months after we started building WebPT in 2006, we had a beta product ready to go; after another 6-8 months of revising and testing, we launched WebPT at the APTA Combined Sections Meeting in February of 2008."

Question: WebPT includes tools for clinical documentation and scheduling, but also coding and billing, and with your relationship with MedBridge therapists have access to continuing education. Did you have a vision for a program this complete at the beginning? What relationships were necessary to bring WebPT to where it is today?

Answer: "Brad and I came up with the idea for WebPT while driving back to Phoenix from Brad's dad's house in Prescott, Arizona. We wrote our ideas about what we envisioned WebPT to be on the back of a bank deposit envelope. To this day, we still have those notes. Early on, our focus was on educating consumers about what PTs did, what diagnoses we treated, and our treatment plans—which is similar to how WebMD started. We also envisioned creating a community where PTs could come to interact and learn from each other. Additionally, we imagined a job board, an e-commerce marketplace where therapists could buy clinic supplies, and, of course, the documentation portal. In evaluating the competition to look at ways we could set ourselves apart, we found that other companies focused heavily on billing. But, no one was doing a good job of providing solid, PT-specific documentation. So, when it came time to narrow our focus, we tackled the biggest problem I was facing: the need to cut my transcription/dictation expenses.

I think people sometimes forget that WebPT started with only our clinical documentation. We weren't always a multi-product platform. In the beginning, we focused on providing therapists with the ability to enter patient demographics, complete SOAP notes, and then fax them to their referring physicians. Essentially, we created a digital patient chart. In doing so, we tackled the biggest pain point that I was having in my own practice—which, as it turns out, resonated with the entire industry. Because back in 2008, 80% of PTs were still using pen and paper. So, even though WebPT was born well before its debut, we didn't have a product we felt was truly launch-ready until 2008.

We built the software with little expectation of it becoming what it is now—at least in the beginning. However, we gained traction early on, and after conducting some market research, we found that we had stumbled into a product with a lot of potential.

Once we figured out that we had something marketable—and that people were willing to pay for it—we launched in the hopes that we could help other clinics improve their operations and bottom lines like I had done.

I think the fact that we didn't go into it with a laser-focus on an exit (e.g., acquisition or IPO)—which is what happens with many software startups—is really what allowed us to grow organically and expand honestly. And that, in turn, helped us stay true to our vision and preserve our company culture—two of the most important ingredients in our success.

As we started to grow, we discovered there were more problems facing therapists and clinic owners that we could help solve. So, we started adding other features and products to our platform.

Eventually, we evolved our vision to be the ultimate software solution for rehab therapists—not just the ultimate EMR.

We wouldn't have been able to grow as quickly as we did without taking on outside investment, but that was something we approached with great care. We were very picky about the investors we ultimately decided to work with, because we wanted to make sure they aligned with our vision.

Our company culture has also been a major ingredient in our recipe for success. It drives everything we do—every decision we make. I believe that our biggest asset is our people, and I think hiring decisions are crucial to any company that's growing rapidly."

Question: Running a software company is not something you learn how to do in PT school. What is the biggest challenge you have faced, and how did you deal with it?

Answer: "One of the biggest challenges I've had to face is the shift in my identity. Before WebPT, 85% of my time was devoted to being a clinician; I spent the other 15% on the administrative activities that come with the logistics of running three clinics. At that time, instant gratification and making an impact on my patients' lives every single day defined my identity. So, when it came time to transition into my role as a business leader 100% of the time at WebPT, I was lost for a while. The transition was difficult. As a side note, I gained a new identity at the same time I was transitioning into my role at WebPT: I became a mother when our daughter, Ava, was born in April of 2011. With all of these changes, I started to understand that I had to shift my focus. When I was a practicing PT, my focus was on my patients and how I could help them improve physically. Now, my focus is on helping my peers, my team, and the industry as a whole achieve greatness—whether that's in PT practice, a career at WebPT, or state and national advocacy forums that push for positive change across the entire industry. My aim is still to help people.

There's also the gender element of being a female in the technology industry. From the time we launched WebPT, I've been the only woman on the executive leadership team, and I was also the only woman on the board until Chelsea Stoner came along with Battery Ventures in 2014. I'm no stranger to being the lone wolf. My experience as an athlete—and the many years I spent working for male sports teams—helped me feel prepared and more comfortable with that type of situation. Still, the tech field was very different from what I was used to in the PT world. So, to effectively navigate this change, I had to adjust the way I carried myself, my tone, the way I approached conversations, and even my body language. It's the little things that have made the biggest difference.

As for WebPT-specific challenges, I think the other biggest challenge has been keeping our culture intact while experiencing massive growth in a short period of time. In an effort to overcome this challenge, we hired a culture captain in 2010 to help foster, focus, and define to our employees what the WebPT culture is and why it's so important."

Question: The reach of the Internet allows tremendous scale. Is WebPT being used in interesting places? How did your message find these locations?

Answer: "WebPT is used all 50 states in the US as well as US territories such as the US Virgin Islands and Guam. I think the most interesting place it's being used is in an animal acupuncture clinic in Oklahoma. It might sound like an odd fit, but it actually makes sense with the way our documentation is laid out. Because vets don't have to worry about billing insurance, they're able to use our therapy-specific format for their own practices. Actually, "animal therapy" is a growing segment of our industry; there is already a special interest group for it, and soon, a certification will be available.

As far as where our customers find our information, they find us online through WebPT's marketing efforts. That can include educational articles on the blog, ads, and features in other online publications. From the very beginning, we have put a lot of emphasis on creating an online community where we could share educational information. We were embracing content marketing before it became a marketing buzzword. Along the way, we've developed a unique voice and tone to help foster that community spirit. For example, we call our customers "members" because we want them to feel like they belong—like they're part of something way bigger than themselves. Just as we want our employees to believe in and get behind our vision, we want to drive the same kind of buy-in among our members, too. Our marketing team does a fantastic job of getting the word out there via our online outlets and social media platforms. They truly highlight what makes us so great and why our members love our product and our community so much."

Question: What goals do you have for your company, and more importantly, when did you come to have them?

Answer: "Our overarching goal as a company—the mission we've always been dedicated to—is empowering rehab therapists to achieve greatness in practice. That has been our rallying cry—the charge that gives meaning to our work and inspires us to put our hearts and souls into doing right by our members every single day. We might not have put words to it in the early days, but the quality of our service and the care with which we delivered it were always of the highest importance. We've always been a customer-centric organization—putting our members first—and we've always placed a lot of emphasis on providing amazing customer service and support.

Now, as for our company goals, we want to continue to build a great business. That means meeting the needs of our customers, staying ahead of the innovation curve and delivering the solutions therapists need—in some cases before they even know they need those solutions. We are committed to staying laser-focused on the rehab industry. I am incredibly passionate about the rehab therapy profession—it's my profession, after all—and this company is my legacy, my way of giving back to the therapy community that has provided me with so much opportunity and joy over the years. And that drives me to keep innovating—to keep pressing forward and pushing the envelope—every single day."

Question: Having a team of skilled people can exponentially increase what can be achieved. How do you know when to add your first employee, or your fifth, or your tenth?

Answer: "In the early days, we would assess our needs, look at our budget, and decide what was the highest priority—another server or another employee? As we've grown, we've become much more sophisticated. Now, we have metrics that drive our hiring decisions. For example, in our billing service team, we know exactly how many claims our team can handle. So, when sales hits the mark and we approach the threshold, we post an opening. We also know how long—on average—it takes to fill an open position, so we time our postings accordingly. As we've become more sophisticated in our processes, our decisions have become much more data-driven.

That being said, we have never strayed from our rule of hiring for culture first and skills second. We look for the candidates that have grit and determination, who are self-starters, and who demonstrate passion and drive throughout the interview process. As we conduct interviews, we try to push candidates out of their comfort zones so we can see past their interview personas and get to know who they really are as people—because that's who is going to show up on day one. I urge other business owners to do the same. Because while you can teach new skills, you can't teach dedication. You can't teach work ethic. And you can't teach passion. We look for the candidates who bring something fresh and new to the table, because when you consciously create a cognitively diverse team, you're going to be more successful. That means when you're ready to hire another employee—whether that's number two or number 200—you'll be confident in your decision to bring that person onto your team. At WebPT, we also fire fast and hire slow. And that means sometimes we're running a lean business. But, that's what's made us who we are today. One of our core values is "Do Mas with Menos," and we hold true to this value when it comes to building our team. When we hire, we don't fill positions just to fill them."

Question: Are you still working as a PT? Does running a software company give you the same fulfillment as treating patients?

Answer: "I recently earned my Doctorate of Physical Therapy (DPT) from Evidence in Motion (EIM), and although I don't officially practice, I seem to have an employee in my office at least once a week asking for some advice for either themselves or a family member—which I love. As far as fulfillment, my role at WebPT has changed my life. I've learned more in the last 10 years than the other 30 combined. I always tell people that I've had an MBA education on the job. To lead the product vision at WebPT, I must stay current on all industry trends, regulations, and innovations. So, while I'm not treating patients, I've found new passion in helping PTs be better in business. Each day, we empower more therapists to achieve greatness, which means they're better able to treat their own patients. And we're still growing, which means we're continuing to provide employment and growth opportunities for so many great people here in the downtown Phoenix area. That's what keeps me going."

Question: Is there anything else you would like to share with readers?

Answer: "I think my biggest piece of advice to therapists and practice owners looking to increase their income and revenue potential is to not be afraid to challenge the status quo. I wouldn't have gotten to where I am today if I hadn't taken a risk and followed my gut instinct. So, if you think you have a great idea, get out of your own way, and pursue it! Even if it doesn't pan out, it's good to get into the entrepreneurial mindset, because it primes your mind to recognize new opportunities as they come along."

Full interview with Heidi Jannenga is available here.

http://bit.ly/26aDghP

Physical Therapy Software Services "Raise the Ceiling" Scores

Required Overhead — Unfavorable to Neutral. Software takes time and skill to code. Most therapists do not have this background. Hiring software engineers is not inexpensive. Developing a minimum viable product, then testing and refining it, can take months and years. A product that has too many bugs and glitches will not be user-friendly enough to get good customer reviews. During a recent episode of Shark Tank, an entrepreneur pitching a software venture was seeking a first round of capital investments of $600,000 just to secure patents and develop proof of concept for an idea that he felt would need another round of investments to reach $1.1 million before profitability could be realized.

Financial Risks — Unfavorable. Lots of money can go into software development, all for a product that isn't used and doesn't sell. All investments are at risk until sufficient traction is gained to reach a tipping point.

Revenue Opportunity — Neutral to Highly Favorable. This depends on the pricing models and the number of customers. The sky's the limit. Overprice your product and it may not sell.

Slowlane vs. Fastlane — 100% Fastlane. Scale provides tremendous leverage within this category.

"Time for Money" vs. Passive Income — Neutral to Highly Favorable. Creating a software product takes considerable time and energy. The first few months or years can be trading time for ***zero money***. Once a product has been developed and is refined, it will still require ongoing updates and users will need support. It is possible to hire additional people to meet these needs, but as a company grows the demands on the leaders will also grow, and at an exponentially higher rate. While perhaps not fully "passive," leaders of software companies multiply their time by the number of people they employ. What can be accomplished by their influence expands tremendously.

Time Frame To Success — Unfavorable to Highly Favorable. It can take years to develop software that is ready to release to the public. Then it has to be sold to users. Once a tipping point is reached—if it ever is—companies can experience explosions in growth.

Long-Term Potential for Increased Income — Neural to Favorable. Not every software program makes money. Not every EMR survives decade after decade. The marketplace is big and there are a lot of software companies in medicine who are looking for opportunities for growth. However, physical therapy has a lot of needs that specialized software can meet, and a well-developed program can have a long life within the profession.

Potential for Sale at Exit — Neutral to Highly Favorable. Does the software make money? If not, then there is nothing to buy, unless they are patented ideas within the software that another company could incorporate into their technology that will help them make money. It is a different story, of course, for successful companies. Acquisition could happen for several reasons. Investors purchase companies to enter into new market space, or to acquire subscribers. Perhaps the software is dated, and a large company wants to sunset the product and gain market share for their own product(s). Perhaps an investor wants to move into a new region of the country, or into a new market segment.

	PT Software - Creation Phase	PT Software - Wide Adoption
Required Overhead	Unfavorable	Neutral
Financial Risks	Unfavorable	Unfavorable
Revenue Opportunity	Neutral	Highly Favorable
Slowlane vs. Fastlane	Fastlane	Fastlane
"Time for Money" vs. Passive Income	Neutral	Highly Favorable
Scale	Highly Favorable	Highly Favorable
Time Frame to Success	Unfavorable	Highly Favorable
Longterm Potential for Increased Income	Neutral	Highly Favorable
Potential for Sale at Exit	Neutral	Highly Favorable

Physical Therapy Product Creation

The final business arena that we will discuss is the creation of new physical therapy products. This involves invention, idea development, sourcing parts and manufacturing, the patent process, audience testing, raising capital, establishing a sales mechanism, marketing, and launching the product.

Everyone loves Shark Tank. There's something thrilling about seeing the work that entrepreneurs have put into products, especially when it makes the sharks go wild. It's even better when the show is a re-run and the Internet serves up success stories of the months after the initial airing. It's equally disheartening when the sharks are tough. There is a strong sense of honesty on the show, and while some entrepreneurs don't get a deal, they get a big dose of real-world business. This reality is there for the physical therapy market, as well. It is a microcosm of the world at-large, and even though we therapists know this market well, we are not given a free pass.

Why develop products for the rehab world? Generally we use products that are on extremes of the spectrum: either very inexpensive and uncomplicated commodities, or very high-priced exercise machines or modality equipment. Yes, therapists can be part of developing anti-gravity systems and force plates for gait analysis and new-fangled e-stim/ultrasound combo units with all the bells and whistles. These products require hundreds of thousands of dollars to develop, if not millions, and this is beyond the reach of practicing PTs who do not have additional funding. The simpler end of the spectrum is easily within reach for therapists. This is where we'll focus our discussion.

Before we go any further, it is important to know that I am not a lawyer, nor an accountant. You should seek business and legal advice for any endeavor you attempt.

It all starts with an idea, or does it? There are two approaches for getting started. One is to look at all the products that are currently used in the physical therapy market, look at the ways therapists work and all of the needs our patients have, and then see gaps in the spectrum of products. Fill the gap, and you could create a product that has tremendous potential. This approach is missing one important element, however: a substantial number of buyers who are ready to purchase.

The second approach is to build an audience or become part of an active social media group of thousands of therapists, and find out what this group wants through your interaction with them. Pitch an idea. If it sticks, then you could have an idea that will work. If it flops, then you'll know not to pour your resources into developing something that will not sell.

Working off of your own spark of inspiration is thrilling and very rewarding. It is business, however, which means there is overhead. No matter how fun it is, if a product doesn't sell then all the time and money invested in development is for nothing (there is learning, of course, but nothing *financial*). Working to meet the needs and wants of an audience can be rewarding, though maybe not as much as following your own spark of inspiration.

Launch day for these two approaches can differ dramatically. Any dullness in the approach of creating a product an audience wants vanishes when strong sales come from that audience during product launch. The thrill of developing your own idea can have a bucket of cold water poured over it if the launch is welcomed by the sound of crickets. Both approaches can have success. Follow your own path, but know that there is more wisdom in spending your time, creative energy, and money developing a product that an audience has already told you they will buy.

Assuming you have an idea, what is the next step? If you don't already know how to make it, you need to talk with people who can help you get started.

In the fall of 2014 I had the idea to create an over-the-door finger ladder. I spent several months looking at product images on Google, hoping to find something already in production that could be repurposed for this task. Plastic ladders, conveyer chain, planter chain, even parrot ladders. Each time I got close, there was something that wouldn't work: either cost, or weight, or both.

Frustrated, I called a few product design companies. Thankfully, they offer a NDA upfront (non-disclosure agreement), or I wouldn't have know to ask for one. A NDA gives inventors some protection from design companies learning of their idea and then taking it to market first. There are several companies across the country that provide a one-stop-shop for all product invention, development, manufacturing, and marketing services. Their price wasn't cheap.

Eventually I learned about freelance designers that offer their services on ELance (now called Upwork). Working off of references, I made arrangements to work with a designer from South Carolina. David was his name. NDA signed, David listened to my idea with interest and immediately thought that my finger ladder idea could be a "cut and sew" product. This was a "eureka" moment—I had never considered cut and sew. So, I found a cut and sew prototype company in Oregon. The gentleman there—his name was Jack—was very helpful and made many suggestions about how to make an over-the-door finger ladder. I gave these ideas back to David, and he worked on a design.

The first drawings came and I was thrilled, but we needed a prototype to be built. It seemed simple enough. Jack was willing to make it, but the product had morphed from cut-and-sew to more of an assembly project—a rope threaded through some ladder rungs and an anchor mechanism, basic parts you could buy at a hardware store. I built one. It took an hour, but I was thrilled. A few attempts later and I had a prototype that was decent.

The Alabama Institute for the Deaf and Blind specializes in production techniques that people with limited vision can perform. They gave me a tour of their plant and looked at my prototype. A few weeks later they gave me a price for assembly. It was high. High enough that it scared me.

In addition to labor costs, material costs were part of the equation. Even though wooden ladder rungs seemed simple, I couldn't find anything that was the right size and shape with pre-cut holes. This would require a custom part. A wood supplier in Illinois gave me a quote that seemed ridiculously high.

Do you see a trend here? I had no idea how much it would cost to have a simple product manufactured. My assumptions were way off.

A friend with experience in the cabinet business recommended that I talk to cabinet manufacturers about sourcing ladder rungs locally. It just so happens there is a cabinet shop that I pass by on my way to work. I stopped in for a visit.

The owner's name is Lee. A savvy businessman and product innovator himself, Lee talked with me about the concept and looked at my current prototype. Fortunately for me, unfortunately for him, he has had multiple shoulder surgeries and went through therapy each time. He immediately understood the benefit that the product could bring. Lee came up with a different approach to the ladder, one that eliminated assembly cost.

Here is an important take home point. Just as there are thousands of ways to take care of a patient, there are many ways to manufacture a product. Designers and engineers are expensive. It is possible to spend thousands of dollars on plans, only to have a manufacturer tell you that there is a better or cheaper way to make a product. Starting with manufacturers to learn their methods and their capabilities and costs and then incorporating those into the design can be a more efficient path to product creation.

One more point about design: manufacturing processes differ greatly in cost. To get the lowest cost per item, it may be necessary to invest thousands of dollars. For instance, plastic injection molding requires a mold. The design and manufacturing of the mold can cost several thousand dollars. If you want to make a small change to your product you will need a new mold. Upfront costs can be substantial, but it may be able to reduce product costs over 50% with high volume orders.

This is not the method I chose. The UELadder is made with a form of computer assisted routing, and the design can be changed any time. We have progressed from prototype to version 1.0, to version 2.0, and now we are evaluating a small change that will be version 2.1, all within six months. This would not be possible with more substantial manufacturing processes. At some point we are certain that our design is finalized, and when there is sufficient volume, we will explore some type of plastic molding.

It didn't take long after our initial meeting, and we had a working prototype in hand. The next few weeks were spent tweaking the design, finding a name, forming a company, designing packaging, finding an assembly plant to package the product, filing a provisional patent, getting liability insurance, and setting up a website. Now it was time to sell.

Let's drill down into a few of these items.

Provisional patents are granted to give inventors a year of protection in which to develop and attempt to sell their product. A full patent application must be filed by the next year or the protection of the provisional patent will be lost. If the patent is granted, then the full patent is retroactively enforced to the date the provisional patent was submitted.

How much does all of this cost? Generally, the fees for filing a patent are not high. The legal work that ensures your patent fully covers your intellectual property can be expensive, though. Fortunately, provisional patents are placeholders for the full patent and are not reviewed. I avoided legal costs, wrote up the provisional patent myself, and paid a filing fee of $130.00. There are many examples of provisional patents and how-tos available on the Internet. Write your application like you would an initial evaluation. It is not that complicated. You have to have drawings that reflect your product, and these came from my designer, David.

When the time comes to file the full patent, seek help from an attorney. Hopefully there will be sufficient sales by then to warrant the few thousand dollars this could cost.

Liability insurance is a definite in healthcare. Finding a company that will give you coverage can be challenging, especially when you are a new company and have a new product. The first price given to me on this was $5,000 per year. Even with no frame of reference, this was still quite shocking. I kept shopping, and eventually found insurance for far less. Typical coverage is $3,000,000 aggregate, $1,000,000 per incident, but you can get less coverage for less money.

Forming a company really isn't that hard. It's far less complicated than completing applications to PT school. The hard part is knowing what type of business structure to choose. There are advantages and disadvantages to all types, which is beyond the scope of this book. When you're ready to form a company you're also ready to find an accountant. Get professional help setting up your company based on your goals and your current situation.

Setting up a website is one of the easier things to do—at least the mechanics of setting it up—but it is the beginning of one of the more difficult parts of the process. There are several e-commerce platforms available. These provide websites, shopping carts, and templates that can be modified as you choose, all for a monthly fee. All of this can be done as an independent site where there will be no recurring fees, but building it can cost anywhere from a few hundred to a few thousand dollars. Amazon is another possibility. They charge a 20% referral fee for the traffic they provide, but it can be worth the price.

Having a website is easy. **Getting traffic is difficult. Converting traffic to sales is challenging. Turning sales into profit** by keeping overhead low and meeting demand is complex.

For every one of the above statements, it is staggering how many books and blogs and instructional resources are available that teach how to do them. A very popular saying about business is, "To get rich in a gold rush, sell shovels." Plenty of online gurus are making millions teaching people how to set up websites and get traffic and sell product. It is possible to spend thousands of dollars on courses and master classes learning what to do. Before spending a large amount on instruction for yourself, consider whether it might be better to spend the same money hiring a specialist to optimize your website and sales material.

What methods are there for getting a therapy product into the marketplace? Who is the end user? Is your product for therapists or for patients? This will determine what tactics to use.

Finding a name can be one of the most challenging things to do. Who are you selling to? Patients? Therapists? For my product, I chose the name UELadder. This may mean nothing to the end user, the patient, but to therapists or doctors who frequently use the "upper extremity" abbreviation, I thought this would give immediate understanding that the product was a therapy tool for the arm. There are patients who seek out finger ladders directly, but just as therapists recommend shoulder pulleys, my assumption was that I would get the most momentum from therapists recommending the UELadder to patients.

As you can see, reaching this point in the journey takes more than a little effort. What happens next can make all the difference in the world.

Tim Ferriss has a blog post that describes how Harry's, a direct marketing razor company, launched their product. One of the founders is quoted as saying, "We couldn't launch to crickets." The post describes how Harry's gathered 100,000 emails in one week and launched to thousands of eager fans.

Another way to reach potential buyers is advertising. Compared to the world marketplace, the therapy industry is tiny. It costs $4,000 per month to get one commercial spot during college football games on ESPN that will only reach the viewers of cable TV in one county. For the same money you can have an ad in 2-3 therapy magazines and reach over half of the therapists in the country. The problem with this approach is that $4,000.00 is a lot of money on a PT salary. And after developing a product for several months it is very easy to have thousands of dollars tied up already.

Marketing alone is not enough. Advertisements need to quickly tell a story of why a product needs to be purchased. Legend has it that the toothpaste company, Pepsodent, had to educate the public on a condition called halitosis, or bad breath, before its toothpaste sales took off. There's a lesson for therapists here, as the promises of clean teeth and decreased cavities weren't compelling reasons for consumers to buy Pepsodent. It's not enough to wave a UELadder in the air and say, "This is a great finger ladder!"

The main selling point of the UELadder is that it can be installed without reaching overhead. This sets it apart from shoulder pulleys—probably the number one HEP tool given to patients with shoulder pain. Isn't it funny that the number one tool we therapists issue for shoulder range of motion has to be installed at the top of a door? Think about it: if a patient can reach overhead, do they need a pulley? Yes, someone else can install it, but, what if that's not an option? Conveying this message quickly and effectively in an advertisement has been not been simple.

Sales efforts for the UELadder have worked. After being in business for just six months, the UELadder has sold all across the country, in twenty-seven states thus far. Patients have purchased the device directly, both through the UELadder website and through Amazon. (Fulfillment By Amazon (FBA) is a service that allows products to have Prime Shipping. It is amazing what a difference this makes for sales.) Some sales have been directly to therapy companies. Pricing is structured so that a clinic could retail the product to their patients and make a 28% profit. This is important, as it gives clinics an incentive to use the product. This doesn't appeal to everyone, as not every clinic sells home exercise supplies.

Distributors like OPTP and Meyers PT are also a good way to sell products, and they are evaluating the UELadder now. It is important to know that distributors ask for significant discounts, in the neighborhood of 30-40% below MSRP. Yes, it will be great if you can move thousands of units with distributors, but products need to be priced in a way that there is profit for all involved—the company, the distributor, and the retailer—at a price point that the end user feels is acceptable.

During my interview with Jarod Carter, he mentioned this experience:

"Once I started looking into making a physical product for hamstring stretching, and I got to the point where it was going to take $25,000 to get the cost down to make enough units to make it worth it [and] I realized: if I do this, I will need $25,000 and all this time. And then I have to find an audience, people to buy it.

Luckily, one of the podcasts I was listening to way back then mentioned someone putting $50,000 into a yoga mat. In the end, he didn't really sell that many of them. He ended up losing all his money.

The proper approach would be to find an audience or build an audience first, then provide them with what they want based on your interactions with them. Luckily, I didn't go down that rabbit hole..."

To help appreciate how building an audience first can help product development, let's follow another physical therapy product through its launch: the Arc.

The Arc was developed by Gene Shirokobrod, DPT, and Corey Fleischer, a mechanical engineer and winner of Discovery Channel's Big Brain Theory. It's a device aimed at aiding posture and providing cervical and lumbar pain relief. Use it by lying in supine position with the device either under the cervical spine or the lumbar spine. Foam pads mimic the feel and pressure of a manual suboccipital release technique.

Enough patients told Gene that they wished they "could take him home" with them that eventually the idea to turn a technique into a product was born. He discussed this with an entrepreneur friend, who connected him with a top-notch designer in Corey Fleischer. Together they developed 3D printed prototypes and began discussions with manufacturers.

Rather than press ahead with an order, the duo took the Arc to Kickstarter. Kickstarter is a crowdfunding platform where newly developed products can be promoted to the public. Those who support the project can "back" it with a pledge. Projects that receive a target number of dollars pledged are "funded," at which time all of the "backers" credit cards are billed for their pledges.

The Arc first went to Kickstarter with a $20,000 target amount, but it only received $12,000 in pledges. Not deterred, Gene and Corey tweaked their plan, initiated some social media marketing, and returned for another attempt. The second time the device was on Kickstarter the Arc surpassed its goal and received total funding of $30,000.00. This afforded Gene and Corey the confidence to move ahead with manufacturing at a much higher level than they could have sans Kickstarter.

Having a successful Kickstarter campaign built a customer base and gave the Arc great exposure. The product and company have been featured several times in newspapers and journals centered in the Baltimore, Maryland area. Current momentum has carried the Arc all across the United States and into multiple countries worldwide.

Q&A with Gene Shirokobrod, DPT

Gene was kind enough to answer a few questions for this book. Here are a few takeaways from our conversation:

Question: Of all the physical therapy products out there, the Arc is one of the few—if not the only one—that was launched with Kickstarter. You even auditioned for Shark Tank! Will you describe the journey?

Answer: "A buddy of mine who is an entrepreneur stayed after me to create something. I told him that I had an idea for a product, and he hooked me up with my partner now, Corey. Corey was on the Discovery Channel show, Big Brain Theory. He's the guy that won—he won the entire show. It turns out he lives 30 minutes from me.

So, we got hooked up, went over to a shop, got a bunch of 3D printers. I told him my idea and he loved the idea of making something that would help people. We 3D printed a bunch of prototypes, and tested it out. Then I found Kickstarter and thought, okay, let's put it on Kickstarter and see what happens.

At that point Kickstarter had a strict no medical device policy. We decided not to think of the arc as a medical device. It's a product that will help people's posture and it's portable, and it will help them feel better. We eliminated anything possibly medical about it in our descriptions, because things like posture are more pop culture and part of everyone's way of life now. It worked. Kickstarter didn't have much issue with it. We were literally the first product, not only in physical therapy but any field straddling that medical line. We were the first product like this that Kickstarter accepted.

Question: Kickstarter is a great place to get crowd funding, but a lot of work has to be done before the campaign begins. How long did your pre-campaign journey take, and what were the big lessons you learned?

Answer: "The pre-campaign wasn't that long because my philosophy was this: I wanted to proof a concept. I wanted to see whether there was a market for this. So, we got everything together, we got the prototypes done, and we just launched. We put it on Kickstarter. The thought process was one, if people really like it, then obviously we'll have a successful product and it'll work on Kickstarter. If not, then, there's no point of even moving forward.

We launched and we ended up raising like, $12,500 in 20 some days, I think, but our goal was $25,000. We didn't hit our goal but we were pretty thrilled because we were able to raise half of it without any marketing. We literally just put it up on Kickstarter and now, this.

The cool thing with Kickstarter, even if you have an unsuccessful Kickstarter campaign, you still have your pay job and you can connect with the people that did pledge. So, we got in touch with them, we found out some things that they liked and didn't like. And then we created another version of arc. This time we did more social media stuff and marketing.

Within four seconds of putting it back on Kickstarter, we had a pledge! A woman told us she was checking every day, seeing when we were going to be back on. In that instance, I knew that we were really good. We ended up getting $30,000 of our $20,000 goal.

The biggest thing is to try to stay away from is paralysis by analysis. You have to go out there and try it."

Question: A product expands your reach far and wide. Has the Arc been purchased by people in interesting locations?

Answer: "At this point, it's kind of crazy. I mean, we have sold it to places you'd never think of: 32 states and 10 countries. We had somebody buy one in Afghanistan that's stationed at one of the US Army bases. All over. All over, countries I've never even heard of.

We started a little map, "Where does the Arc go." It's cool having something people can buy anywhere and just go all over. But the craziest place...I still think it's crazy that somebody in Afghanistan in an Army base is using an Arc. To me, that's awesome."

Question: Finding inspiration for a therapy product might not be too difficult for therapists, but working to create a viable product company is very different. How did you learn how to do this, and where can therapists go to get more information? What books are resources do you recommend to aspiring PT entrepreneurs?

Answer: "That's a tough question. Even when you're successful—whatever success is to you—it's tough because there's so much you have to figure out, from manufacturing to shipping. International shipping is a real pain. You just go through ups and downs. We've been a company for about two years and I think I already been burned out twice.

The best thing you can do is just to get a foundational understanding of how to set up those systems to run when things are going well—not just when they're going poorly, but when they are going well and investing in that.

Where you can go to learn that? That's the beauty of it. That's the cool part. It's everywhere. You can go online and look at best practices for businesses, and there's blogs, and there's a lot of cool books that you can just Google on Amazon and go buy, or a course or things like that. That's what I did."

Question: If there is one take home message about developing a product that stands about the rest, what would that be?

Answer: "My take home message is that it's very much analogous to just running a business where you have ebbs and flows. It's not about your product, it's about the perception of what it'll do for the people in the audience. And the biggest takeaway is you have to scale the connection to your audience. It's taking that physical therapy perspective of a one-to-one and combining to thousands, and hundreds of thousands of people, and then selling that.

In terms of crafting the message, I think the best thing is using your physical therapy knowledge because—I say this all the time—physical therapists are the worst best sellers, I think, in the world. We're clinically trained to get people to say yes, you know? But if you can integrate that, if you can move past the roadblock that you're trying to sell something to make money, then I think you start to really think like your audience. That has helped me the most."

Full interview with Gene Shirokobrod is available here.

http://bit.ly/264XJrY

Physical Therapy Products "Raise the Ceiling" Scores

Required Overhead — Unfavorable to Favorable. Startup costs can easily reach tens of thousands of dollars. Once a product has a modicum of success the overhead to run a product company can be low.

Financial Risks — Unfavorable to Favorable. This depends on scale. While you can get started with just a few thousand dollars, many products fail. If you choose wisely in what you develop and find creative ways to launch, a few thousand dollars is all you need to get started. The bigger the market, the bigger the company; the bigger your launch, the more upfront money will be needed and the more is at risk.

Revenue Opportunity — Neutral to Highly Favorable. This depends on the pricing models and the number of sales. The sky's the limit. Overprice your product and it may not sell. Develop a product that customers love and promote, and you'll have explosive growth.

Slowlane vs. Fastlane — 100% Fastlane. Scale provides tremendous leverage within this category.

"Time for Money" vs. Passive Income — Neutral to Highly Favorable. Creating a physical product takes considerable time and energy, as does finding an audience and marketing, as well as developing a supply chain. The first few months or years can be trading time for ***zero money***. Once a product is established, it will still require ongoing marketing, and users will need customer and sales support. It is possible to hire additional people to meet these needs, but as a company grows the demands on the leaders will also grow, and at an exponentially higher rate. While perhaps not fully "passive," leaders of product companies multiply their time by the number of units they sell. What can be accomplished by their influence expands tremendously.

Time Frame To Success — Unfavorable to Highly Favorable. It can take months and years to develop a product that is ready to release to the public. Then it has to be sold. Once a tipping point is reached—if it ever is—product companies can experience explosions in growth.

Long-Term Potential for Increased Income — Neutral to Highly Favorable. Not every product makes money. Plenty of ideas tank. The marketplace is big, and there are a lot of product companies in medicine who are looking for opportunities. Miss your patent and your idea could be stolen. Competing products can creep into your space and steal away market share. There are no guarantees, and all the rules of free enterprise apply. That being said, some products generate strong profits for many years. Developers of one product establish distribution channels and, over time, usually develop multiple products.

Potential for Sale at Exit — Neutral to Highly Favorable. Unsuccessful products have no value unless patented ideas within them can be incorporated into other products. Successful products with widespread utilization and substantial annual sales can have very high multiples, perhaps as high as twenty or more.

	PT Product Creation and Early Growth	PT Product Wide Spread Adoption and Utilization
Required Overhead	Unfavorable	Neutral
Financial Risks	Unfavorable	Unfavorable
Revenue Opportunity	Neutral	Highly Favorable
Slowlane vs. Fastlane	Fastlane	Fastlane
"Time for Money" vs. Passive Income	Neutral	Highly Favorable
Scale	Highly Favorable	Highly Favorable
Time Frame to Success	Unfavorable	Highly Favorable
Longterm Potential for Increased Income	Neutral	Highly Favorable
Potential for Sale at Exit	Neutral	Highly Favorable

****

Reminder —
- *P*ut your affirmations & visions in your head and heart.
- *T*rack your progress with journaling.
- *C*hallenge your status quo.
- *S*hare your journey with a friend and colleague.
- *G*row: read, listen, and watch to develop new skills.

"Let today be the day you give up who you've been for who you can become." —Hal Elrod

****

Part 5

Conclusion

Chapter 15

Concluding Thoughts and Parting Business Advice

"For which of you, intending to build a tower, does not sit down first and count the cost, whether he has enough to finish it"
—*Luke 14:28*

Physical therapy as a profession has many, many strengths. In today's economy it is incredibly valuable to be able to quickly get a good-paying job anywhere you want. Providing care to those in need is tremendously rewarding, and interacting with people can be more interesting than interacting with equipment or computers or designs. PT is a noble career path, and one that is respected by all. What's more, it can be a launching pad for growth into many different fields, interests, or business pursuits.

What was a huge strength twenty years ago—that the healthcare sector was always strong even when other industries failed—is not proving to be as true today. Physical therapy is affected by the winds of change within medicine, and the trend of rising costs and decreasing reimbursement is cause for concern. Unless a major shift occurs within healthcare as a whole, therapists' salaries will likely stay flatlined or diminish over time, while volume expectations and documentation requirements will increase. Elevated demands and diminished rewards can lead to frustration and burnout.

Are therapists loyal to such a noble profession bound to accept limited potential for increased pay because the healthcare environment that surrounds us is changing? The answer is yes, if we stay within our comfort zone and only seek to be employed during normal business hours. Are therapists who innovate and find ways to expand their means less noble because they achieve elevated income? No, not at all. In fact, when these therapists benefit the PT community by employing other therapists or by providing educational services or products that are needed and used, they earn much deserved admiration and respect from their peers. Their reach and impact on patients is far greater through the reach of others than they could ever achieve on their own.

What risks are we willing to take? With almost every business model we discussed there are financial risks. Some have strong potential for the present, but limited potential for exponential growth. Others have no ceiling, but a huge barrier to entry in upfront costs and energy.

There is another financial risk that we didn't discuss at length, and that is the risk of doing nothing. By taking no action we risk missing opportunities.

If we continue to do what we have always done, it is almost certain that we will get what we have always gotten. To take this path and hope for a different result is what Albert Einstein called "insanity."

Greg Todd recently posted a video blog about this very topic. Here is how he summarizes the clip:

"Let's face it...one of the things that draws many of us to start a career in PT is that there is pretty solid stability in the field. There is basically a job around every corner. It might not necessarily be something you like, but you can pretty much find a gig somewhere if you're desperate enough. You can't really say that for most professions.

Sometimes that's a good thing...but sometimes that can create a lack of urgency.

Today on my video blog   (http://youtu.be/1jEfNl34HYg) I talked about a story in which I and another physical therapist got the same opportunity to work with top-level professional tennis players and I took it and he didn't... He felt like it was just too inconvenient to work after normal work hours.

Because I took that opportunity, my career took a completely different path than his.

He's had five different jobs during the time that this one opportunity led me to start my business and grow it to what it is today.

If there's one thing I can tell you, it is that you need to have a sense of urgency in anything that's really important to you. If you are looking to make more and do more than the average PT, you really need to understand this concept."

One of the first steps we need to take in moving forward is to examine our own heart and determine our own passion. As so many therapists interviewed in this book have said, striving for higher income only for the sake of getting more money is not a good reason. Is it possible to feel the limitations of being employed and wish for the freedom that others enjoy as a result of taking a different path without wishing for higher income? Perhaps not. Burnout and frustration have a significant self-centered component to them, which can create an attitude of wanting to get rather than give. MJ DeMarco said that wealth affords three things: health, time with friends and family, and freedom. These are noble goals, though still somewhat self-serving.

Income is a direct result of the effect we have on the world, and the size of that effect for each person we touch. Within the spectrum of professionals in healthcare, surgeons are able to affect the greatest change in the shortest amount of time for their patients. Therapists affect great change, as well, but these results come over weeks and months. The natural result, of course, is that surgeons receive a much greater monetary reward for their work. Therapists can earn higher incomes than surgeons, but only by affecting many, many lives.

Therapists who treat with their hands alone make a difference in thousands and tens of thousands of patients over their career. Therapists who hire therapists multiply their impact by five, twenty, one hundred—however many therapists are under their employ. Therapists who teach impact hundreds of thousands of lives through the efforts of their students (though they typically are not rewarded monetarily for this impact). Therapists who develop software and products apply their skill to create the tools therapists use, and by their talents give aide to the masses.

If therapists who want to avoid or break through an income ceiling can expand their ability to give, then this can expand their means.

Within physical therapy, Fastlane strategies not only provide wealth, but they also make it possible to exponentially increase impact for patients and other therapists alike. This latter goal, if it is our true motivation, will be respected by all, and more importantly, will act as a compass for our businesses. Profits will be needed because businesses are in business to stay in business. As a business grows, the rewards provided to the owner grow as well, both in income and in the satisfaction of knowing you are making a contribution to so many people.

Before we reach the very end and close out this "episode of care" with a Discharge Summary, I have one more section of wisdom to share. At the end of a lot of interviews I asked if there was any advice to share about income ceilings and starting a business. Here are their responses:

Advice on Starting Your Own Business

Jarod Carter, DPT, of DrJarodCarter.com

Question: What advice do you have for physical therapists who have hit the income ceiling, and who look at what you are doing and think they want to start a business of their own?

Answer: "It's very easy to look at the business you're working for and look at the total revenue in terms of what you're generating per patient and think that your employer must be making a ton of money. And if you just do it on your own, within a year, you'll be taking your own huge percentage of all that revenue. You will need to take a closer look at what overhead costs would be if you have never owned a business. And then double that, just to be safe. There's a reason why a twenty-five percent profit margin for a brick and mortar business is enormous.

In terms of running your own brick and mortar business, your own practice, if you never had a business, you really don't need to underestimate the amount of overhead you're going to have. Definitely save six months of expenses. Avoid debt if you can.

You also want to consider your time and what's important to you. If you have a growing family and you're not ready for twelve, fourteen hours a day for the next potentially a year or two, at least... You have to factor that in before you make that leap. Some people find a quick and early success, but for a lot of people, it really is a grind for a while. I don't want anyone out there thinking that if they just hang out the shingle it's going to happen almost on its own, and then kick themselves for not really taking stock of everything that's going to go into it, not just financially but also time-wise.

When you do that, if you still have a passion for starting your own practice, it needs to be because you have a passion to be your own boss, not just make more money. I think that's an important distinction, as well. If you really don't have to be your own boss but you're just hoping to make more money, I think that you'll find better avenues than starting your own private practice.

Similarly when you hear about online business owners who have fast success and are making a ton money people can mistakenly think it all happens very quickly without a ton of work. There are people that are able to make crazy, amazing stuff happened quickly without too much work, but in general, that doesn't happen. It does take a ton of time to set it all up.

Try to build an audience first. You might have an idea, a product—whether it's physical or a media product—but before you really start working hard on that product, make sure there is a demand for what you're creating. You can spend a lot of time creating something that, if no one asked for it, then no one is going to buy.

Another thing I wish I had focused on earlier is having a systems-based mindset, and documenting all the things that you find that worked, and then tweaking those documents as you improve those procedures and systems. If you document things along the way, you can let your staff or your team have those notes so they can do exactly what they're doing. Then you can scale so much faster when you want to bring someone on. You have the video, you have that task list ready for them. So, as you go, no matter what business you're in, document those systems, what works, and what you find yourself repeatedly doing. And then, delegate. Get it off your plate."

Aaron LeBauer, DPT of LeBauer Consulting

Question: What advice do you have for someone who might look at your success and think that they might want to start either a cash-based practice or an online business?

Answer: "You have to know why you want to do it. Know what your motivation is and be real, and be genuine in communication with people and your marketing. Don't let anyone tell you that you can't do it or it's not possible because if I listened to these people, then we wouldn't be talking right now."

Karen Litzy, DPT, host of the Healthy, Wealthy & Smart Podcast (on iTunes)

Question: I'm sure it's still work, but reading your website seems like your job is so much fun. What advice do you have for therapists who have hit an income ceiling, who look at your story and think that they want to get outside of the box and start their own business?

Answer: I think it's all about the individual, your individual situation, but there are lots of ways to make extra money. I mean, if you just did a bit of the side hustle, like I did for many years. I live in New York City and it's very expensive. The salary of a PT alone just didn't cut it. I would say a good majority of my friends that are physical therapists here in the city see patients on the side on their own because you have to. This is New York, you know, you got to hustle.

If you feel like you've hit the ceiling, I think that there's definitely other ways to get yourself out there. Some people will hook up with a home agency, which can pay very well, depending on the area, or you can get yourself out there and start your own thing. I did an online seminar last year for physical therapists to do just that. And I've had emails from physical therapists saying, you know, I went through module one of your seminar and I did everything that they said to do, here's my website. I'm starting my business. So, it's not that hard if you have the right tools to do it. And I think you just have to be smart, you have to be proactive, you have to read a lot.

I think you need a good lawyer. I say this every time someone asks me. You need a good lawyer, you need a good accountant. Anybody can create an LLC or PLC, or some sort of corporation, whatever entity works for you. On the side, you just do it. Start going out and meeting people.

The biggest thing you have to do is you have to know why you're doing what you're doing.

And if the only reason you're doing what you're doing is to make money, then maybe that's not the right reason. If you're only doing it for the money, then people are going to see right through that. I mean, you're not gonna get any referrals, I can tell you that.

But if you're doing it because you love what you do and you're trying to expand your reach, and you want to reach more people, and you're coming from a give-to-get mindset, then I think you'll do very well.

Myra Bolton Scott, OT/R, President of Champion, Partners in Rehab

Question: What advice do you have for therapists who look at what you are doing and think to themselves that they want start their own business?

Answer: "I've really always tell people that I had to take a risk and leave a very secure job to do what I do. It was something that I had to think long and hard about. My faith was involved and I prayed about it.

So, I don't try to discourage people from taking that leap even when it feels scary because you've got to be willing to get out of your comfort zone if it's something you really want to pursue.

But I also try to encourage people to be really honest about what they perceive as their strengths. And, again, just because you're a great clinician with very creative patient care ideas, that's not going to necessarily make you a successful owner of a company. Really look at what do you want to spend your days doing. Are you going to miss being hands-on all day? I knew I wasn't gonna miss that. I always enjoy the success of the patients as a sum total of all the therapists that were working with me.

There are a lot of therapists out there with a lot of good skills, and a lot of them that could be very successful, but I think they're held back by fear sometimes.

I think the other thing I would tell is that I don't think anybody builds something big by themselves. It takes having the right people around you. You know, Champion certainly would not be Champion had I not been given some of the opportunities I've been given and had I not had some of the people that I've worked with. So, it's never…it's never "all me." It covers a lot more when you do work as a team.

You need a partner whose strengths balance yours. I have to say that where I needed the most help, those were the areas of my business partner's strength. I told him from the beginning I don't know a thing about payroll and taxes. I don't know a thing about getting the political system to fight for a Certificate of Need. The combination has been a good, and I don't think we would be near successful had I not had that partnership. So, he is due a lot of credit."

Tom Pennington, PT, CEO of Physician Rehab Services

Question: Do you have any advice for therapists who look at your success and think that they want to start their own therapy company?

Answer: Yes, I do have some advice for therapists that want to start and own their own company. First of all, I feel like success should never be defined in financial terms. I think that is one of the last definitions in success. Look at success as defining your passion and then finding a way to work within that passion in a meaningful way that brings purpose to you and those around you. This can be done certainly in physical therapy, and it could be done if you cut grass or picked up garbage. Those that are passionate about something and work hard in it more times than not find a way to make the finances work. I used to define financial success that if I could order a pizza on Friday without balancing my checkbook, it was a pretty good week. I personally have never been motivated by the dollar, but certainly am pleased when it's there when you need it.

With that said, my advice to therapists wanting to start their own company is to realize that whenever you start something on your own that it will require sacrifice, and that it will fully permeate your life, as well as the life of your family. For instance, if I ever work for someone again, when I get that paycheck and take it to the bank, I will have a new appreciation of what it took for that money to be in the bank at the time I cashed that check. I will also have a greater appreciation for any benefits that I will receive from the company, because I realize they come at a substantial cost and effort. There have been times when we have paid employees and not paid ourselves. There have been times when our line of credit was fully used, and we might be facing a $400,000 payroll with $30,000 in the bank. I think that if any business owner is honest, he/she will tell you that there have been times of fear, times of rejoicing, times of hitting your head on your desk and thinking "Why in the world have I gotten into this?" I think that the person that is getting ready to embark on this needs to be fully aware of the risk, the commitments, and the sacrifices. I think they really need to a gut check to see if they have the risk tolerance and the drive to make the emotional sacrifice.

I have a great amount of respect for my barber who 40 years ago converted an old two-bedroom house into an 8-chair barber business, an old school business where you come in, sit down, and whoever calls you up cuts your hair that day. I asked him one day his philosophy on business, and he said, "Tom, you just have to will it to happen. This doesn't look like much, but when I bought this old house years ago it was a second mortgage. I didn't really know how I was going to pay for it. I used it to cut hair and rent out on a monthly basis the additional chair space. I got good people as barbers to help me so that things would work out." Indeed for Jim they did work out. I've thought about his advice many times, because I think to be a success and to be viable, you just have to will it to happen, sometimes over and over and over."

Sean Sumner, DPT, Best-Selling Author of Sciatica: Low Back Relief Once and For All

Question: What advice do you have for therapists who have hit the income ceiling, who might look at what you are doing and think they might want to write a book to supplement their income?

Answer: "I would tell people to go for it. I do believe there is an income ceiling and that's why I've done this. I know that for the work that I want to do in physical therapy there is an income ceiling that I'm going to meet, if I haven't got close to it already. I'm the lead physical therapist in my unit, and if I want to make more money I need to go into management, and that's more of a time commitment, and really not that much more money. I know that's not what I want to do in my life — I love treating patients. I like the work that I do but I want to be able to have more money for my family and for myself. Writing books, to me, is not only the best way of earning more, it's the easiest way to do it. You'll get a return quickly. You can spend three months, then the book can be out. It's passive income. I can't stress that enough. You can always get other jobs. I've picked up shifts in fitness facilities, in hospitals and all those things. And you can get other positions that make more money if you want, but you only have to much time. With passive income in books on Kindle, that money comes back to you and it's not something you have to devote more and more hours to every time you want more money. You write a book and you market it well and it's passive income that comes in that is not taking more time away from you."

Mike Reinold, DPT of MikeReinold.com

Question: What advice do you have for physical therapists out there who have hit the income ceiling, who might look at what you are doing and think to themselves that they want to start an online business?

Answer: "Starting an online educational platform is a lot of work. You need to be passionate about it to be consistent."

Eric Gartner, DPT, Co-Founder of SimpleSet.net

Question: What advice do you have for therapists who have hit an income ceiling, who might look at what you are doing and think that they want to start a software business?

Answer: "Starting a small business (software or otherwise) should be to solve a problem you are passionate about. Starting a business with only a monetary goal in mind is probably not a great idea. In the early stages of any start-up, money is going to be nonexistent or very tight. If you don't have a passion for your idea, it will be easy to lose focus and pack it in. Chase what you are passionate about and money will inevitably follow. With a bit of hard work and luck, a side business can end up generating an income that can help you break through any financial ceiling you run into, and it can be a very satisfying experience."

Heidi Jannenga, DPT, Founder and President of WebPT

Question: What advice do you have for therapists who have hit an income ceiling, who might look at what you are doing and think that they might want to start a software company?

Answer: "When providers reach a wall in growing their income, I encourage them to think outside the box. That said, I firmly believe that doing things solely to make more money will not lead to success. For me, I wanted to work with Brad to create a software solution that could help solve a problem plaguing my clinic. And while we worked together, I continued to work full time treating patients and full time building a software solution—with no guarantees on what the outcome would be. Building your own business—especially a software business—isn't easy. It's hard work, and we spent many nights asking ourselves if it was really worth the stress, angst, and financial strain. But, when you have a passion for something and start to experience some traction, it keeps you going. It's very much the same as treating patients. You try some treatment methods that may not work at first, but when you adjust your approach and start to make a true difference in someone's life, it motivates you to keep going and to come into work everyday. And I get to experience that level of motivation on a daily basis—from my peers in the PT industry as well as with my team at WebPT.

It's like crack—I'm addicted! I really just want to keep pushing forward to see our vision become reality. Now, I understand not everyone is going to create a software from scratch. In fact, that's probably not the right route for many people. But, I encourage anyone with the entrepreneurial itch to evaluate what they're already doing and challenge themselves to be innovative, whether that's embracing direct access, adopting new technologies, offering different types of products or services (think cash-based), or expanding their marketing efforts. Furthermore, don't settle for the status quo: keep iterating and changing based on the needs of your primary customer—your patients."

DISCHARGE SUMMARY

Over the course of a few hours, the reader has been instructed in the reality of salaries within the profession of physical therapy, in the internal and external forces that shape salary levels, and in several business models that are available to all physical therapists that can expand both impact and salaries. Some business models have high risks, some have high rewards. Some rely heavily on therapist man-hours. Others are built on scalable platforms and provide passive income. With this understanding, therapists can evaluate a path for business and anticipate its potential to provide income at a desired level.

The reader has been given a Home Exercise Program, including a 30-Day challenge, and is encouraged to continue to perform these new daily routines and to communicate with colleagues frequently about professional growth and to stay connected with the _The Physical Therapy Business & Entrepreneur Accelerator Community_ well into the future.
http://www.facebook.com/groups/PTBizAccelerator/

Much work awaits anyone who wants to expand their impact by going into business on their own. While the details of forming a business, choosing a tax structure, developing a product or service, creating marketing materials, and selling yourself and your brand are beyond the scope of this book, the general concepts that will determine a business's potential performance have been covered. Therapists are encouraged to seek professional counsel from attorneys and accountants. Most importantly, therapists are encouraged to measure their own passions and life situation carefully ("why") to determine whether or not they have the resources of knowledge, time, money, energy, and family support ("how") to pursue greater professional growth and business developments ("what").

Thank you for reading this book! Remember, greater income is directly tied to greater impact. Have a vision, turn it into reality, and enjoy the wealth of expanded contribution!

May God bless you and the lives you touch as a physical therapist!

"Therefore whoever hears these sayings of Mine, and does them, I will liken him to a wise man who built his house on the rock: and the rain descended, the floods came, and the winds blew and beat on that house; and it did not fall, for it was founded on the rock." —Luke 7:24-25

Full Interviews and Five-Year Growth Plan References Available at
www.UELadder.com/pages/bonus-materials.

Interviewee Resource Links
Jarod Carter
- Medicare and Cash-Pay Physical Therapy
- My Cash Based Practice

Aaron LeBauer
- Cash PT Toolkit
- Cash PT Blueprint

Karen Litzy
- Healthy Wealthy & Smart Podcast
- Creating and Building Your Physical Therapy Practice Course

Mike Reinold
- Blog
- Inner Circle

Lenny Macrina
- Courses Available on Medbridge

Greg Todd
- Physical Therapy Builder

Ben Fung
- Updoc Media Blog

Eric Gartner
- SimpleSet

Heidi Jannenga
- WebPT

Products Mentioned
UELadder
The arc

Full Interviews
Jarod Carter
Aaron LeBauer
Karen Litzy
Myra Bolton Scott
Tom Pennington
Mike Reinold
Lenny Macrina
Sean Sumner
Eric Gartner
Heidi Jannenga
Gene Shirokobrod

Full Interviews and Five-Year Growth Plan References Available at
www.UELadder.com/pages/bonus-materials.

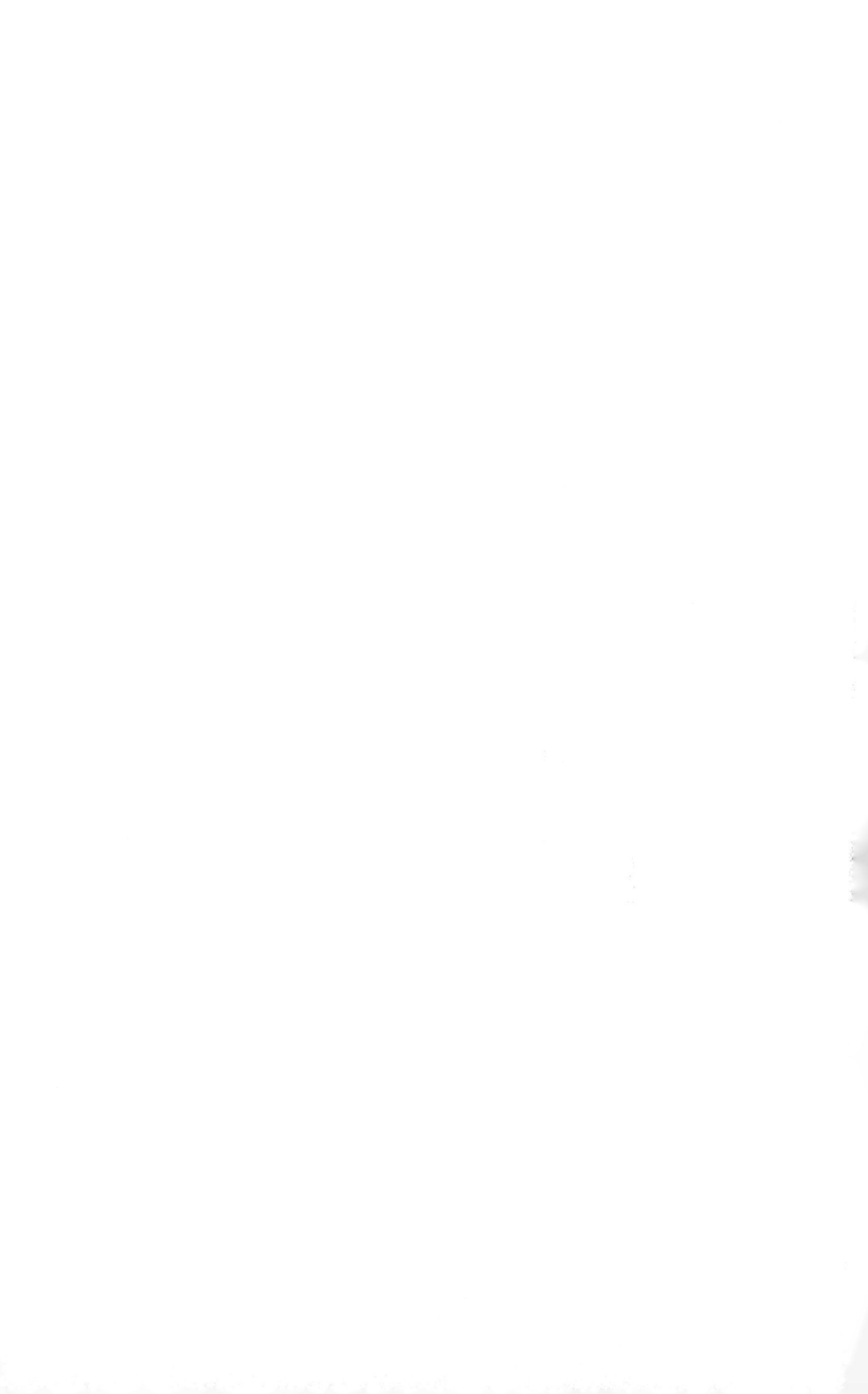

Made in the USA
San Bernardino, CA
15 February 2017